Diseases of Pacific Coast Conifers

Robert F. Scharpf, Technical Coordinator,
Retired Project Leader, Forest Disease Research

USDA Forest Service
Pacific Southwest Research Station
Albany, CA

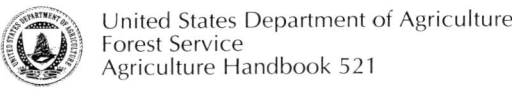

United States Department of Agriculture
Forest Service
Agriculture Handbook 521

Revised June 1993

DISEASES OF PACIFIC COAST CONIFERS
Robert F. Scharpf

U.S. Department of Agriculture
Forest Service

Agriculture Handbook No. 521

Abstract

Scharpf, Robert F., tech. coord. 1993. Diseases of Pacific Coast Conifers. Agric. Handb. 521. Washington, DC: U.S. Department of Agriculture, Forest Service. 199 p.

This handbook provides basic information needed to identify the common diseases of Pacific Coast conifers. Hosts, distribution, disease cycles, and identifying characteristics are described for more than 150 diseases, including cankers, diebacks, galls, rusts, needle diseases, root diseases, mistletoes, and rots. Diseases in which abiotic factors are involved are also described. For some groups of diseases, a descriptive key to field identification is included.

Oxford: 44/#5—1747 Coniferae (79)
Keywords: Diagnosis, abiotic diseases, needle diseases, cankers, dieback, galls, rusts, mistletoes, root diseases, rots.

Contents

Preface iv
Acknowledgments iv
Introduction v

CHAPTER 1 Abiotic Diseases 1

CHAPTER 2 Needle Diseases 33

CHAPTER 3 Cankers, Diebacks, and Galls 61

CHAPTER 4 Rusts 83

CHAPTER 5 Mistletoes 112

CHAPTER 6 Root Diseases 136

CHAPTER 7 Rots 150

Glossary 181
Index to Host Plants, With Scientific Equivalents 188
Index to Disease Causal Agents 191

For sale by the U.S. Government Printing Office
Superintendent of Documents, Mail Stop: SSOP, Washington, DC 20402-9328
ISBN 0-16-041765-1

Preface

This publication is a major revision of U.S. Department of Agriculture Handbook 521, first issued in 1978 and slightly revised and reissued in 1979. It has been updated to include new information that will help identify many of the diseases of conifers growing along the Pacific Coast of western North America. The revisions have been made mainly to provide the latest information on diagnosis, nomenclature, and new diseases, and to expand the coverage of important diseases of the Pacific Northwest. The basic format of this handbook remains essentially the same as the original version. The expanded coverage, more and better illustrations, and new information are designed to make this handbook a useful tool in diagnosing diseases of Pacific Coast conifers.

Acknowledgments

We want to thank our many colleagues who willingly contributed their time and effort to the revision of this handbook. Special thanks go to those who provided photographs, critically reviewed the manuscript, and suggested improvement for use by field personnel.

Dave Adams	California Department of Forestry
Brenda Callan	Canadian Forestry Research Centre, BC Canada
Tom Chase	South Dakota State University
Fields Cobb	University of California, Berkeley
Greg Filip	Oregon State University
Everett Hansen	Oregon State University
Jack Marshall	California Department of Forestry
Art McCain	University of California at Berkeley (retired)
J. R. Parmeter, Jr	University of California at Berkeley (retired)
Jack Sutherland	Canadian Forestry Research Centre, BC Canada
Tim Tidwell	California Department of Forestry
Francis Uecker	USDA Agricultural Research Service, Beltsville, MD

Personnel of the USDA Forest Service

Jim Byler	John Kleijunas
Greg DeNitto	Bill Otrosina
Susan Frankel	John Pronos
Don Goheen	Mark Schultz
Frank G. Hawksworth	Jane Taylor

Introduction
Robert F. Scharpf and Robert V. Bega

Tree diseases are a natural part of the forest ecosystem. For the most part, the native diseases occur at endemic levels and only occasionally appear as spectacular or damaging epidemic outbreaks. However, even at endemic levels, damage to western forests from some diseases can, over time, be quite serious. A few introduced foreign diseases also occur in western North America, and some cause serious injury to native species.

This handbook was designed to bring under one cover the basic information needed to identify some of the common diseases of Pacific Coast conifers. Although written primarily to help identify conifer diseases of the Pacific Coast states, the handbook should be useful throughout western North America where most of these diseases also occur. Diseases of seedlings or of conifers grown in nurseries are not covered in this handbook. Other publications deal specifically with seedling diseases.

The information contained in this handbook is intended to serve a comparatively broad group interested in such activities as resource management, conservation, forestry, tree farming, outdoor recreation, and growing ornamental trees. Except for a few texts written on forest pathology, most of the available literature on tree diseases is in the form of bulletins, monographs, articles, and shorter contributions issued from time to time through a variety of publication outlets.

A tree disease is primarily a disturbance of the normal functions of a tree or the deterioration of its parts. Therefore, it is fundamental to recognize the parts of the tree that are attacked by disease-producing agents and the kinds of disease common to them. Also, when attempting to diagnose a particular conifer disorder, the environmental conditions that allow disease-causing agents to adapt and successfully attack must be kept in mind. The roots of a tree, for example, require conditions for infection and establishment of an organism widely different from those to be found surrounding the leaves of the same tree. An organism causing a disease of living tissues may possess a different mode of attack and environment than one that produces a heart rot in the dead tissues of the heartwood.

AGENTS OF TREE DISEASE

Agents of disease can readily be classified as (1) **abiotic**, non-organic, nonliving agents, such as air and soil pollutants, ice, snow, wind, frost; and (2) **biotic** or living organisms, such as mistletoes, bacteria, and fungi. Viruses are not included because they have not been found to cause diseases of western conifers.

Climate, soils, and vegetation vary greatly along the Pacific Coast. The cool, humid conditions of the Pacific Northwest contrast with the arid conditions of southern California. Aside from host specificity and biologic competition, the important factors influencing the prevalence and virulence of disease pests are environmental; they include temperature, moisture, soil condition, and human influences. The same disease may, and usually does, have different degrees of intensity depending on the locale and the conditions under which the host is growing. For example, the canker fungus *Botryophaeria ribis* has never been found attacking the giant redwood in its natural habitat. However, when the tree is planted in the warmer areas of western United States, *B. ribis* causes severe branch flagging, top dieback, and even death.

The activities of humans affect most of the diseases described in this publication and must be considered in diagnosing a disease and evaluating the damage caused. On sites where trees are growing, every effort should be made to minimize environmental changes. Logging and construction work— particularly road construction and land leveling for housing, for campgrounds, and for picnic site development—are frequently a source of injury to trees. Apart from mechanical damage to above-ground parts of trees by machinery, roots can be injured if they are severed or if they are covered with excessive amounts of soil. Overdevelopment in previously undeveloped areas may damage trees. Trees may also be damaged in indirect ways, such as through groundwater depletion or pollution.

Conversely, humans must also be protected from diseased trees in recreation sites—particularly campgrounds, picnic areas, and summer home sites. Control of hazardous trees is of prime importance in both existing and future sites. Trees that fail because of disease or other agents can destroy lives and property.

This publication is organized primarily for use in field diagnosis and, except for the chapters on rusts and mistletoes, it describes symptoms based on the part of the tree attacked. Host genus and species are used as a major separation of cankers, mistletoes, and rusts.

Pertinent literature citations relating to the diseases follow each chapter, and a glossary of terms and an index of hosts and diseases are included at the end of this handbook. Scientific names that have become widely accepted since the previous edition are included where appropriate.

Control recommendations are not discussed except in special instances because of the continual changes in methods and materials used for control. As the environment undergoes changes, and as tree values continue to increase, particularly for recreational and esthetic use, specific control recommendations will also change.

DIAGNOSIS OF TREE DISEASE

Diagnosis of plant diseases is the art of identifying a disease from its symptoms, signs, and patterns. The symptoms (expressions of the diseased host), signs (evidences of the cause), and patterns of occurrence provide the clues on which the investigator bases the diagnosis.

The following guide will help diagnose tree disease:

1. Determine as accurately as possible the part of the plant that is actually affected. For example, the death of only 1-year's needles indicates a needle disease; of scattered whole branches—a canker disease; of the whole tree—a root disease, drought, or fire. Note the pattern of the disease in the trees. Is the damage limited to the south side, the lower crown, or the upper crown?

2. Note what species are affected. Are there any individuals that are affected less or that are free of the problem? Also note the condition of adjacent plants.

3. Note the pattern of occurrence. On what areas are the problems most severe? How do these areas differ from those areas free of the problem? Are these problem areas in any particular environmental zone or related to a particular cultural activity?

4. If the cause of the disease is not immediately evident, look first for the simplest effects, such as animal damage, frost, lightning, other climatic influences, simple injuries, fire, or other obvious causes of the problem.

5. Look for the presence of fungi, insects, or other parasites. Observe accurately and try to judge whether the organisms found are the main cause of the trouble or just secondary. For example, insects will frequently move in as secondary causes of trouble on trees weakened by disease.

6. If the whole tree is dead or suffering and nothing is found above ground to indicate the cause of the disease, expose the roots and root crown for examination.

7. If you are still unsure, learn about the recent history of the problem and the area. Is the problem of recent origin, and when was it first noticed? What cultural practices have been carried on in the area, such as the use of herbicides, fertilizers, irrigation or flooding, road salting, and air pollution? Do local weather records indicate the recent occurrence of any unusually severe conditions?

DESCRIPTIVE KEYS

The descriptive keys found in some chapters are based on the host and the causal agent. In each key, letters are followed by either a letter for alternatives or for the causal agent that fits the specimen. Thus, each step leads to another step and its alternatives, until the name of an organism is reached. Success in diagnosing a specimen by these keys depends largely on an understanding of the characteristics used. In many cases, this publication illustrates the key characteristics. If at any point in the key you are undecided about the way to proceed, follow through on the alternatives and compare the disease condition with illustrations and descriptions found in the text or in the references cited.

An example is the key on rots:

- A^1 On incense-cedar, juniper, or redwood .... B
- B^1 On incense-cedar C
- C^1 A brown pocket dry rot (pocket dry rot) .... *Oligoporus amarus*
- C^2 A white stringy root or butt rot (annosus root and butt rot) .... *Heterobasidion annosum*

SELECTED REFERENCES

Cordell, Charles E. [and others] tech. coords. 1989. Forest nursery pests. Agric. Handb. 680. Washington, DC: U.S. Department of Agriculture. 184 p.

Finck, Kelly E.; Humphreys, Patricia; Hawkins, Graham V. 1990. Field guide to pests of managed forests in British Columbia. Joint Publication 16. Victoria, B.C.: Forestry Canada and B.C. Ministry of Forests. 188 p.

Hagle, Susan K.; Tunnock, Scott; Gibson, Kenneth E.; Gilligan, Carma J. 1987. Field guide to diseases and insect pests of Idaho and Montana forests. Missoula, MT: U.S. Department of Agriculture, Forest Service and State and Private Forestry. 123 p.

Hamm, Philip B.; Campbell, Sally J.; Hansen, Everett M., eds. 1990. Growing healthy seedlings: identification and management of pests in Northwest forest nurseries. Special publication 19. Corvallis, OR: Forest Research Laboratory, Oregon State University. 110 p.

Holsten, Edward H.; Werner, Richard A.; Laurent, Thomas H. 1980. Insects and diseases of Alaskan forests. Alaska Region Rep. 75. Juneau, AK: U.S. Department of Agriculture, Forest Service. 187 p.

Sinclair, Wayne A.; Lyon, Howard H.; Johnson, Warren T. 1987. Diseases of trees and shrubs. Ithaca, NY, and London: Cornell University Press. 574 p.

CHAPTER 1   Abiotic Diseases

Paul R. Miller
Plant Pathologist, Pacific Southwest Research Station, Forest Service, U.S. Department of Agriculture, Riverside, CA

INTRODUCTION

Diagnosis of diseases and injuries caused by abiotic factors must take into account the environmental history of trees at a given location. This history includes the varying influences of solar radiation, temperature, water, atmospheric gases, pest or weed control chemicals, wind, fire, topography, geologic substratum, soil, and management activities. Individual causes of abiotic disease or injury may act in an instant (lightning or fire), during one or more seasons (temperature extremes and water deficiency), or continuously over the life span of the tree (geologic substratum or soil). For example, frost can cause injury in a few hours, salt toxicity near roadways occurs continuously during one or more seasons, and the toxicity of serpentine soils is always present. Abiotic factors may exert direct effects singly, simultaneously, or sequentially with respect to one another. Trees may be predisposed to infectious diseases or insect attack following injury or stress by abiotic factors.

The diagnostic evidence of injury and disease caused by abiotic factors is present at the site as symptoms on needles, twigs, branches, main stems, and roots, or as a feature of the landscape surrounding damaged trees. In certain situations, it is useful to consult recent weather records for evidence of temperature extremes, precipitation deficiencies, and gale-force winds. Valuable information can be gained by questioning residents and local forest managers about recent events or management practices.

The visible symptoms that indicate abiotic injury can be categorized according to presence on the main stem, branches, twigs, and needles. The part of the crown affected, including the upper and lower halves and also the inner and outer portions (branch tips), should always be noted as one of the first steps of the diagnostic process.

LOW TEMPERATURES

Winter killing, winter injury

Needles, buds, and twigs—Winter-killed needles are usually completely brown regardless of age (fig. 1-1a); however, tissues at the base of needles may remain green in less severe cases of injury

Figure 1-1— *Monterey x knobcone pine severely injured by below-freezing temperature in midwinter (**a**). Ponderosa pine with less severe injury confined to needle tips (**b**).*

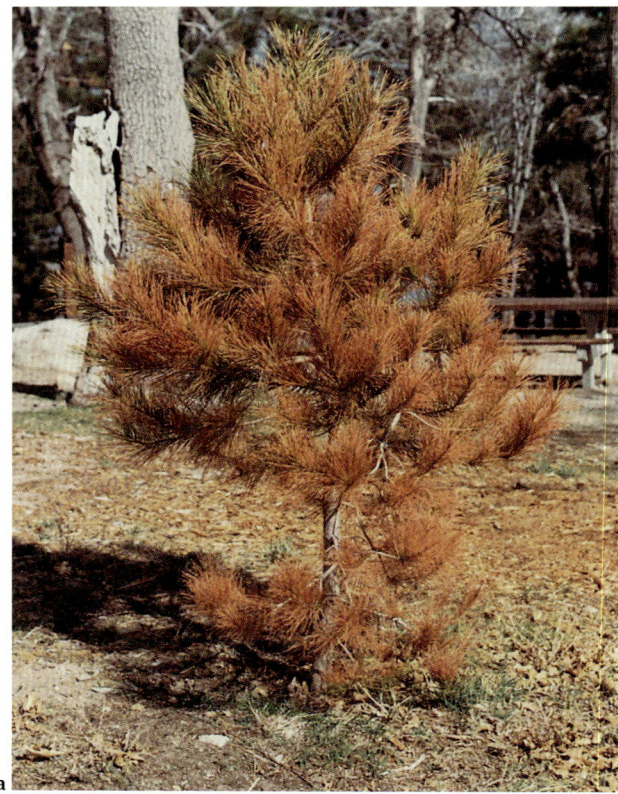

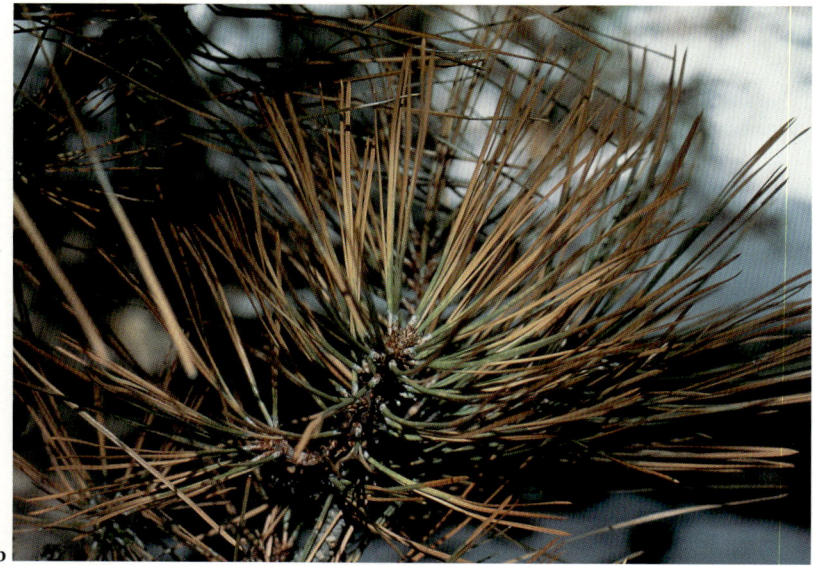

(fig. 1-1b). Discrete brown flecks commonly occur, mainly on the upper needle surface, and show greatest intensity on older needles exposed to the sky and snow deposition (fig. 1-2a,b). Minimum temperatures ranging from –31 to –45 °F (–38 to –49 °C) caused extensive damage to ponderosa and Jeffrey pine east of the Sierra

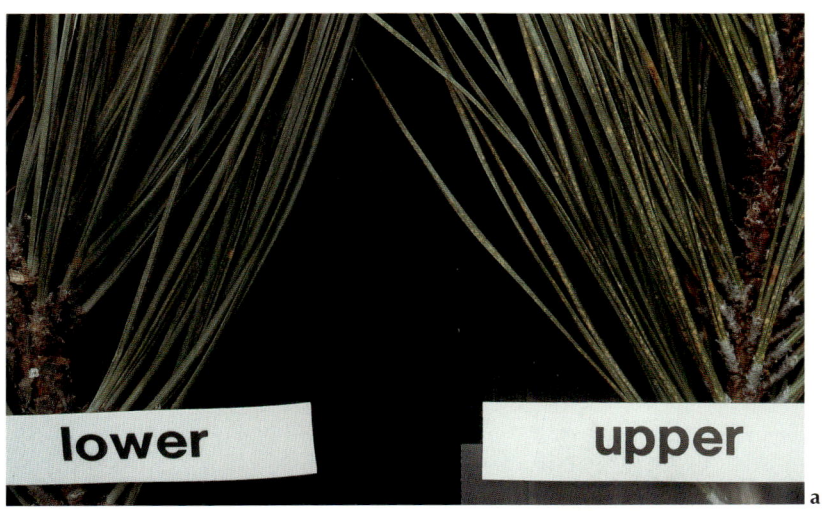

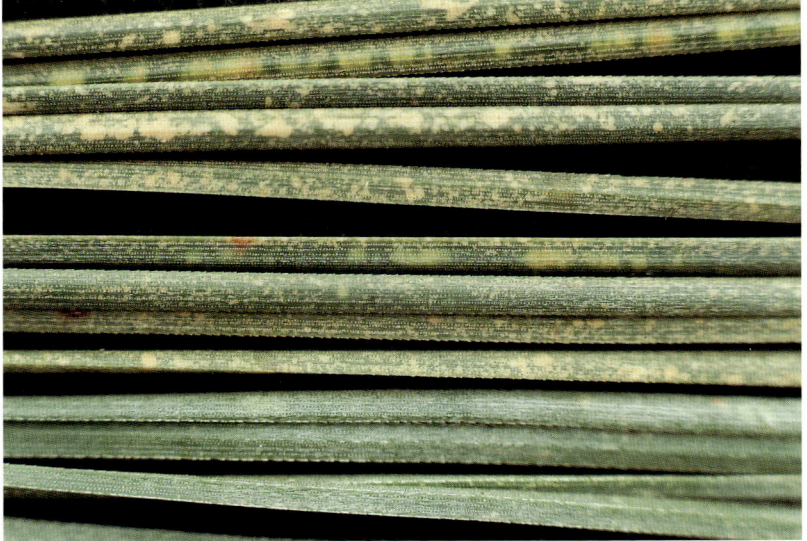

Figure 1-2—*Discrete necrotic flecks on the upper surface of ponderosa pine needles are associated with winter conditions only, particularly snow deposition; lower surfaces of needles show no symptoms (**a**). A close view of ponderosa pine needles from the same tree shows a variety of symptoms ranging from a combination of necrotic flecks and chlorotic mottle on the top and middle to healthy needles on the bottom (**b**). The chlorotic mottle is caused by chronic exposure to ozone.*

Nevada crest. However, affected trees recovered if the inner bark tissues of the main stem were not injured.

The severity of low-temperature injury varies between species and within a species; for example, ponderosa pine was injured more than Douglas-fir during midwinter low-temperature episodes in eastern Washington and differences in injury have been observed among white fir seedlings depending on seed source. Needles of coast redwood seedlings were injured during an 8-day period when the temperature remained between 21 and 30 °F (–5 and –1 °C). Inland plantings of Monterey pine, especially those above the 1,500 feet (457 m) elevation, in southern California were badly damaged when temperatures remained below freezing for several hours during 1 or 2 consecutive days.

Top kill—Death of tops of conifers can occur when a quick drop in temperature follows an abnormally warm period in the winter. For example, top kill of Coulter pines in southern California resulted from freezing of inner bark tissue down to about 5 inches (13 cm) in diameter when a quick drop in temperature to approximately 20 °F (–7 °C) followed an abnormally warm period of 11 days; this particular damage is often called spiketop. Similar injury has been observed on ponderosa pine in northern California. Spiketop may also be caused by drought, lightning, bark beetle attack, defoliating insects, or mistletoe infestation (fig. 1-3).

Frost crack—During periods of sudden cooling, the wood cylinder shrinks more in a tangential than a radial direction, resulting in cracks that usually do not extend more than 20 feet (6 m) up the trunk from the ground. Callus tissue forms over the surface of the crack in the first year. The crack is split and healed again successively through the seasons until it heals completely. Frost cracks are often the source of a watery exudation from the bole of white fir. This exudate is often called slimeflux. Large callus growths that project some distance out from the normal circumference of the trunk are called frostribs. Frost cracks are frequent in older white fir trees, particularly those on the east slope of the Sierra Nevada, and on grand fir in northern Idaho and Montana.

Frosts in spring and autumn

The tolerance of foliage, small branches, and main stems to cold temperature depends on "hardiness," which in turn is closely correlated with the time of year. Low temperatures above freezing and short photoperiods induce frost hardiness. The changes in plant cells associated with frost hardiness include increases in both osmotic pressure and cell protein content. Freezing injury is most often caused by formation of ice crystals within the cell and less frequently by dehydration of tissue by extracellular formation of ice crystals.

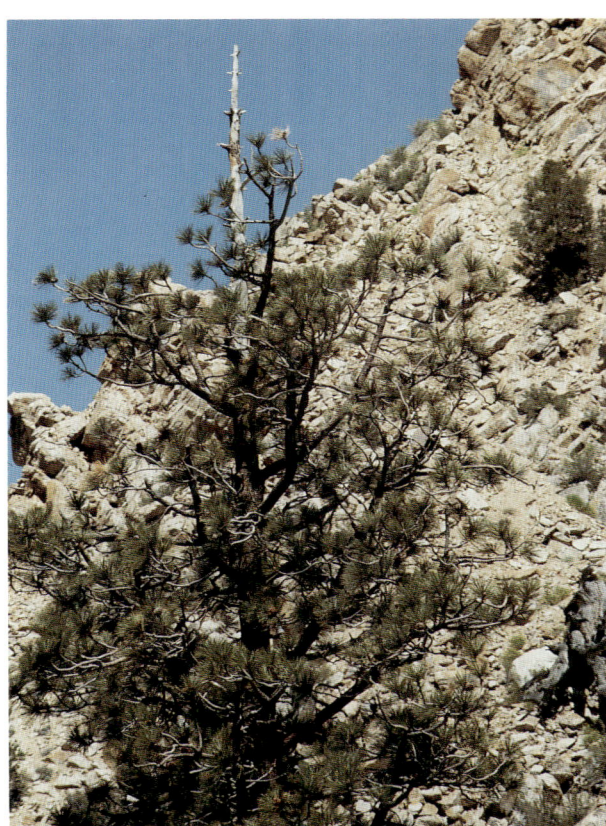

Figure 1-3—*Top kill of Jeffrey pine associated with low temperature. Similar spiketop appearance may be caused by drought, lightning, insects, or mistletoe.*

Increases in osmotic pressure and cell protein content may inhibit intracellular formation of ice crystals. The sudden occurrence of below-freezing temperatures (frosts) in spring or early autumn can severely damage unhardened tissues, actually killing young shoots and needles.

Autumn frost injury—Any succulent shoot tips and current-year needles will be injured if growth is still in progress. A partial list of California conifers in order of increasing frost sensitivity includes lodgepole pine, Jeffrey pine, ponderosa pine, incense-cedar, sugar pine, and white fir. Recovery can be expected the following spring.

Frost lesions form on the main stems of small Douglas-fir as a result of a sudden drop in temperature in unhardened tissues. Later, the sapwood is exposed when the dead bark tissue cracks and falls off. Eventually the lesion is calloused over, but in the meantime decay fungi may enter the area.

Spring frost injury—Spring frost causes differing amounts of damage to conifers, depending on the stage of growth and develop-

Figure 1-4—
Frost-injured white fir in spring show dead young shoots and needles. The shoots and needles will remain on the tree through summer.

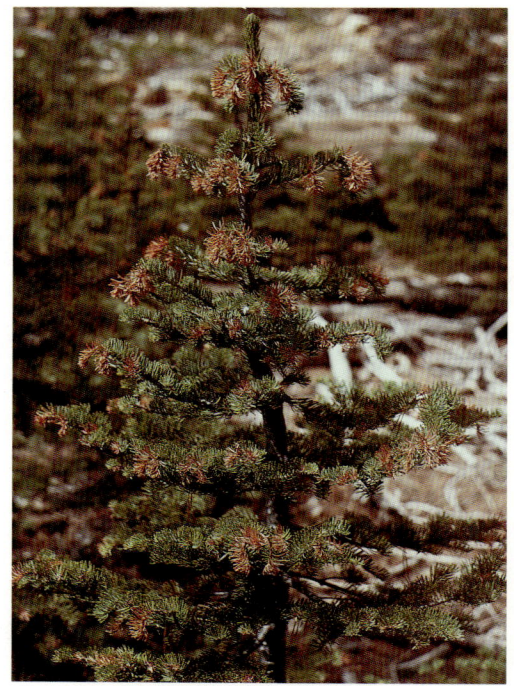

Figure 1-5—
Repeated frost injury to bishop pine planted out of its natural range results in numerous dead branches and ragged tree crowns.

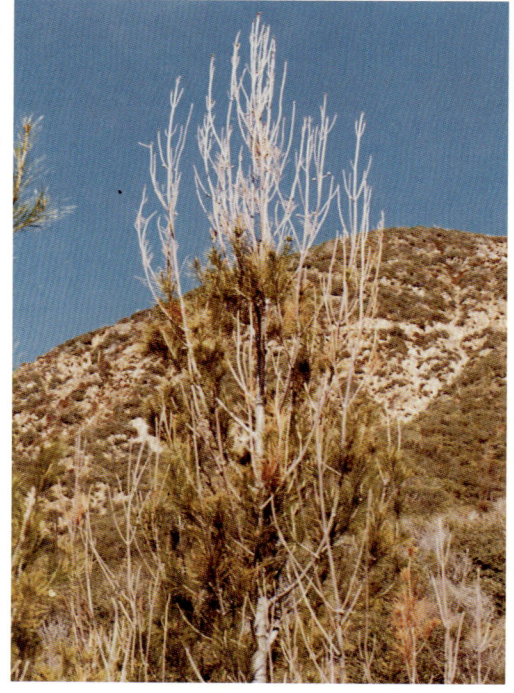

ment at the time of injury. Before bud break, some buds may be killed. After bud break, new leaves and soft succulent shoots usually are damaged. The brown, dead portions usually remain on the tree, and the tree produces new shoots (fig. 1-4). Trees that are repeatedly injured by frosts are characterized by long, dead, main stems with dense growth of needles developing at the bases, forming a bushy appearance (fig. 1-5). Frost injury that is not severe enough to cause death of succulent tissue often results in crooked shoots. Spring frost injury varies considerably, even on the same species, depending on the stage of development of the new tissue. For example, the more advanced growth at the lower elevational range of a species would suffer greater injury than the less advanced growth at the upper limits of a species' range.

An abrupt temperature drop to 13 °F (–10 °C) in mid-April in New Mexico injured the following conifers in order of increasing sensitivity: alligator juniper, Douglas-fir, ponderosa pine, white fir, and limber pine. Limber pine, which was at its lower elevational range, showed the most severe damage because its growth was the most advanced.

Both spring and autumn frost injury are likely to be localized where topographic depressions cause the pooling of cold air; these areas are called frost pockets.

Winter temperature, sunlight, and wind interactions

Red belt—Red belt is so called because of the appearance of afflicted trees distributed in well-defined bands varying from less than 20 to as much as 1,000 yards (18 to 914 m) wide on slopes and benches. Variable lengths of tree crowns display reddish-colored needles that were killed when an unseasonably warm winter temperature was followed immediately by a sudden decrease (fig. 1-6).

Usually, valley bottoms and adjacent slopes are constantly exposed to cold air. The sudden occurrence of warm, dry winds (foehns, Chinook, or Mono winds) produces a temperature inversion, a relatively thin layer of warm air that cannot mix downward and continues to contact side-slopes, at various elevations depending on the time of day. At night, cold air draining down the slopes fills the valley and raises the warm air layer above its daytime level. Trees exposed to unseasonably warm air by day receive cold air at night. This alternation of warm and cold air exposure, along with the frozen condition of the soil, results in desiccation injury because daytime transpiration removes moisture from the needles more rapidly than it can be replaced by roots in frozen soil. Older needles fall off, leaving only current-year needles on living branches.

Winter drying or sun scorch—When bright sunny days follow a period of below-freezing temperatures, several western conifer

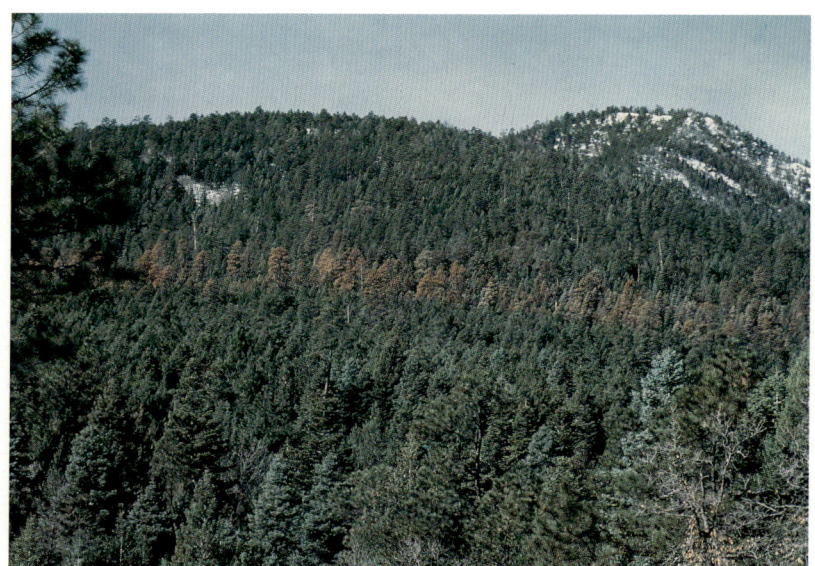

Figure 1-6—Red belt results from injury by excessively cold night temperatures alternating with warm day temperatures. The distinct belt results from the day–night fluctuation of the height of cold and warm air where these distinct air layers contact the hillslope.

Figure 1-7—Young shoots and needles of Jeffrey pine, particularly those on the sunny side, have been desiccated. This occurred during sunny, warm winter days when roots and stems were too cold to transport adequate water.

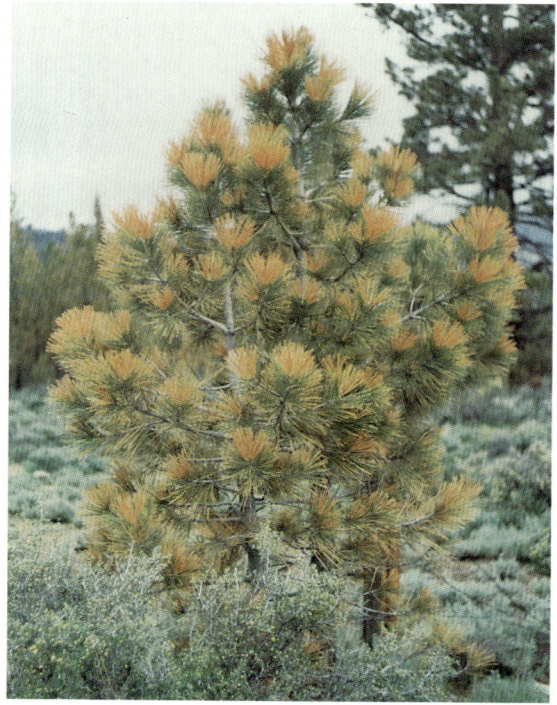

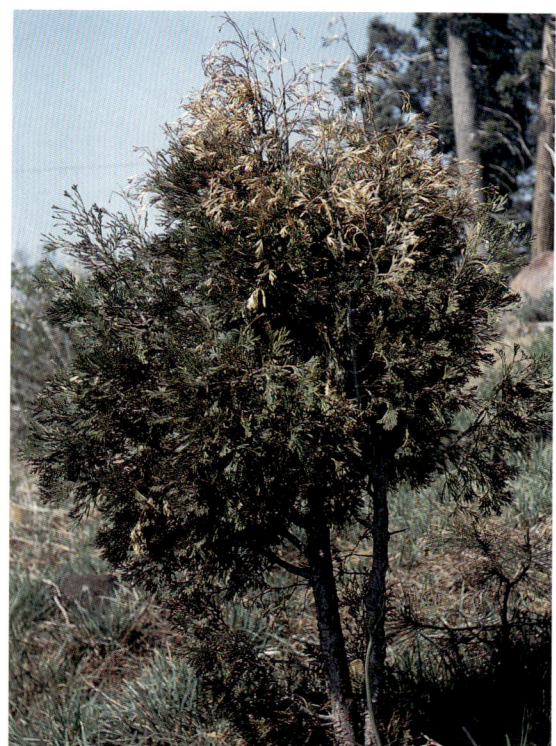

Figure 1-8—Incense-cedar with an unusual bushy form because of repeated desiccation of the top not protected by snow.

species—typically western redcedar—experience conditions causing the leader and several of the youngest branch whorls to die. Usually the south, southeast, or southwest sides of mostly small trees on the border of denser stands, or sometimes the entire exposed crown of isolated trees, show reddish-brown needles (fig. 1-7). Lower portions of the crown where needles are covered with snow never show injury.

The localization of injury on the sunny side of the trees suggests that rapid thawing of sap in the needles in the bright sun and subsequent transpiration without replacement of water (because the roots and bole are very cold or frozen) cause irreversible desiccation of the needles. After repeated incidents, the more sensitive species such as lowland grand fir and incense-cedar will develop a bushy appearance (fig. 1-8). Limber pines at high elevation sites near the timberline have a permanent prostrate form because of continuous injury to new growth (fig. 1-9).

For Engelmann spruce and subalpine fir at the timberline in Wyoming, the windward needles had lower water contents and xylem pressure potentials and more desiccation injury compared to leeward needles. Needle injury decreased with height above the

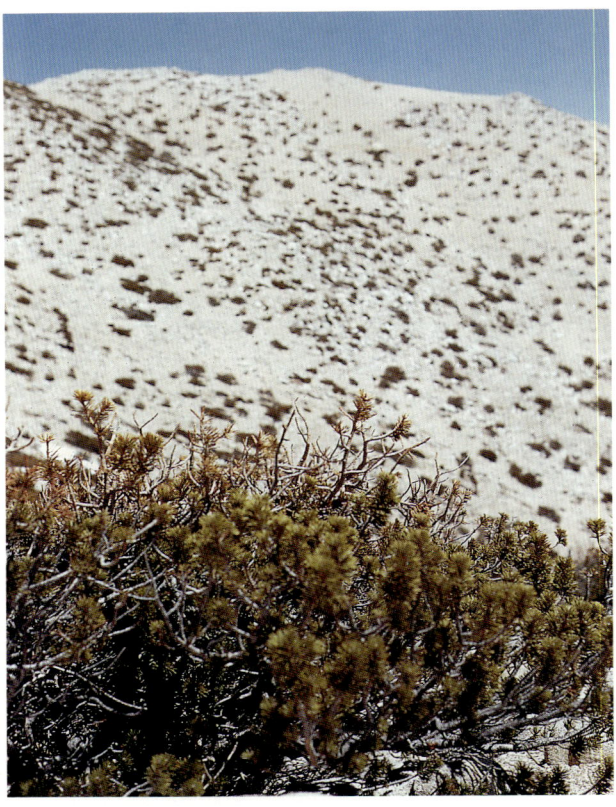

Figure 1-9—*Prostrate growth of this limber pine near timberline was caused by repeated freezing and desiccation of upper needles and branches not protected by snow.*

snow. Probably abrasion of the cuticle of needles near the snowline by blowing snow was responsible for the low cuticular resistance to water loss. Injury to needles below the snow's surface was minimal.

Parch blight—Brief episodes of Chinook winds, the dry winter winds originating east of the Cascade Mountains, occur occasionally in western Washington and Oregon. During these episodes the needles on the eastern edge of single exposed Douglas-fir trees and on the eastern edge of stands may be killed. Even the previous year's shoots may be killed. Although the soil is not frozen, transpiration losses apparently exceed the water absorption possible by roots in cold soil. Injured trees recover almost completely by the following summer. In tests of Douglas-fir seed from 40 provenances, trees from Colorado, Arizona, and New Mexico had the highest winter drought resistance, whereas those from the coastal regions of the Pacific Northwest had the lowest resistance.

Major canopy damage from the combined effects of snow, wind, and winter drought occurs in western North American forests at roughly 9- to 16-year intervals. A single season's events may reduce foliage biomass as much as 42 percent. Stand productivity is reduced in an episodic, largely unpredictable manner.

Minor effects of low winter temperatures

Winter yellows—One of the least harmful effects of cool winter temperatures is the winter yellowing or chlorosis of conifer needles. A breakdown of chlorophyll begins with the first frost; foliage exposed to direct sunlight shows the most severe symptoms, namely, a brassy yellow green color. Giant sequoia often turns a bronze color. The chlorophyll content is restored, and the needles become green after the first weeks of warm weather in spring.

Purple top—Ponderosa pines and western white pines grown in exposed nursery beds show a purple discoloration of the youngest foliage. The tops may eventually become brown and die; surviving seedlings have a bushy appearance.

Necrotic fleck—Discreet tan flecks only on needle surfaces facing skyward commonly occur on conifers throughout western North America (fig. 1-2b). Histological evidence has eliminated fungi as a cause and implicated low temperatures. Circumstantial evidence suggested that exposure to snow is a prerequisite for injury to develop. Flecks are most numerous on the oldest needles but do not seem to contribute to early senescence.

HIGH TEMPERATURES AND SOLAR RADIATION

Needle scorch

Leaves or needles that develop under cool conditions may be injured by sudden temperature increases. For example, needle tip browning results during the latter part of a generally cool spring on coast redwood, Monterey pine, and juniper when temperatures suddenly reach 100 °F (38 °C).

Shoot tip dieback

The developing shoots of Douglas-fir and white fir are particularly sensitive to sudden rises in temperature in May and early June. This injury may be confused with spring frost damage because the shoot tips droop, turn red-brown, and later break off.

The effects of prolonged high temperatures during spring, summer, and fall, in conjunction with soil moisture deficiency and dry winds, may result in extensive top dieback in large trees of several species (fig. 1-3). This condition resembles bark beetle damage, but lack of beetle galleries and the involvement of firs, incense-cedar, and pines together disqualify insects as the cause.

Figure 1-10—
Water-stressed needles of this ponderosa pine have bent at the end of the fascicle wrap where tissue is soft and immature.

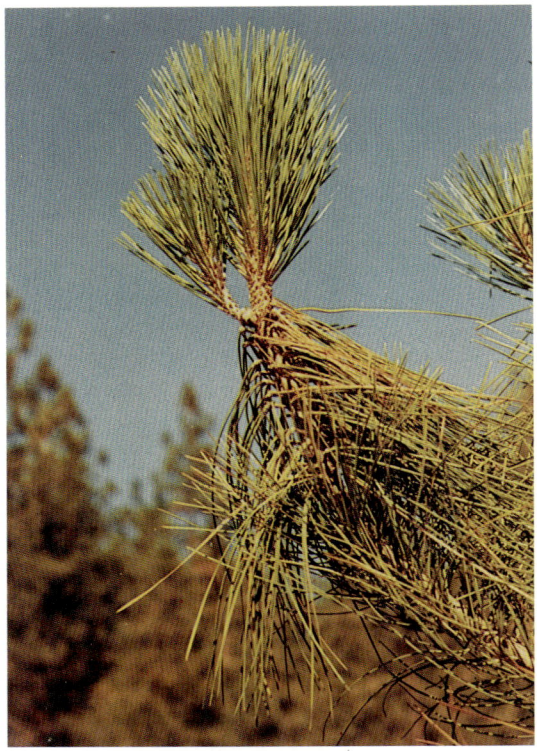

Needle droop

Sudden and excessively rapid transpiration may result in abrupt needle droop caused by collapse of tissues near the base of young developing needles. This condition may be followed by death of mature, current-year needles. The condition is observed on pines in California (fig. 1-10).

Heat canker or bark scorch

On rare occasions, cankers develop on the southwest sides of the main stems of young western white pine, Douglas-fir, spruces, and true firs during the first few years after the stand is thinned. In Douglas-fir, there is a yellowish to reddish discoloration followed by a slight sinking of bark tissue. Later, the bark cracks and scales off. The lesions generally heal very slowly.

An apparently benign effect of high air temperature is sap exudation by needles of Douglas-fir, reported in eastern Washington. Sugar accumulation on needle surfaces and subsequent growth of sooty mold fungi on needle surfaces are commonly observed on conifers infested by aphids.

SOIL MOISTURE DEFICIENCY
Drought

Soil-drought conditions usually develop first on gravels and sands, which hold very little water, and shallow soils overlaying rock or gravel. For this reason, drought-damaged trees usually occur in groups. Conifers that are undergoing only moderate moisture stress will shed older needles prematurely—and often also suffer dieback of needle tips and small twigs. Under more severe stress the needles of the leader and upper branch whorls turn light tan, with the discoloration advancing from the tip to base of each needle, first as a narrow band of yellow, then tan. Drought stress symptoms progress in the crown from the top down and the outside in. The symptoms remaining on surviving trees in subsequent years include dead tops, fewer needle whorls, and shortened needles in the whorls formed after the drought year. The growth of trees that survive drought is retarded. With some conifers, reduced diameter and height growth appear 1 year after the drought. Generally, seedlings and saplings are more severely affected and often die because they have less extensive root systems than larger trees.

During severe drought conditions in California in 1929 and 1960, Douglas-fir and incense-cedar were killed or injured on poorer sites, but ponderosa pine, sugar pine, and white fir on the same poor sites were less seriously affected. During the 7-year drought in the West from 1986 to 1992, pines and true firs died in large numbers from the combination of drought stress and bark beetle attack. Small incense-cedar and Douglas-fir were the first to show drought symptoms. Western white pine were more seriously affected by drought than nearby Douglas-fir and lodgepole pine. Italian stone pine, Aleppo pine, Italian cypress, and Arizona cypress were highly drought tolerant; Jeffrey and Coulter pines were slightly drought tolerant; and Monterey pine was not drought tolerant in comparative tests. Knobcone pine, Torrey pine, single-leaf pinyon, and Digger pine successfully occupy dry sites.

Pole blight

This disease was confined to pole-sized western white pine north of the Clearwater River drainage in the Idaho Panhandle and extending northward into parts of Montana, Washington, and British Columbia. It has not been a serious problem since the 1960's, but it is included here to illustrate the symptoms that might be expected from chronic drought conditions. Affected trees occur randomly first, later in limited patches. The first evidence of injury is decreased radial growth followed by reduced leader and branch growth. Older needles drop, and remaining needles become short and yellow.

The disease spreads downward and inward until the whole crown is affected. Resinous stem lesions appear as flattened areas on the stem.

After extended dry and warm weather, western white pine does not regenerate rootlets fast enough to replace those lost due to moisture stress. The decline of the crown is a secondary reaction reflecting the effects of a degenerated root system. Trees growing on the dry sites, that is, those with low capacities to store soil moisture, are susceptible to pole blight.

EXCESS SOIL MOISTURE

Damage by excess soil moisture is confined to specific sites. Problems occur along the shoreline of new reservoirs or beaver ponds and along new river channels formed by flooding (fig. 1-11) and near highway embankments that impede normal drainage and thus cause the water table to rise.

Overwatering of conifers in ornamental plantings is a common problem that is more severe on poorly drained and poorly aerated clay soils than on sandy soils. Native conifers growing in newly

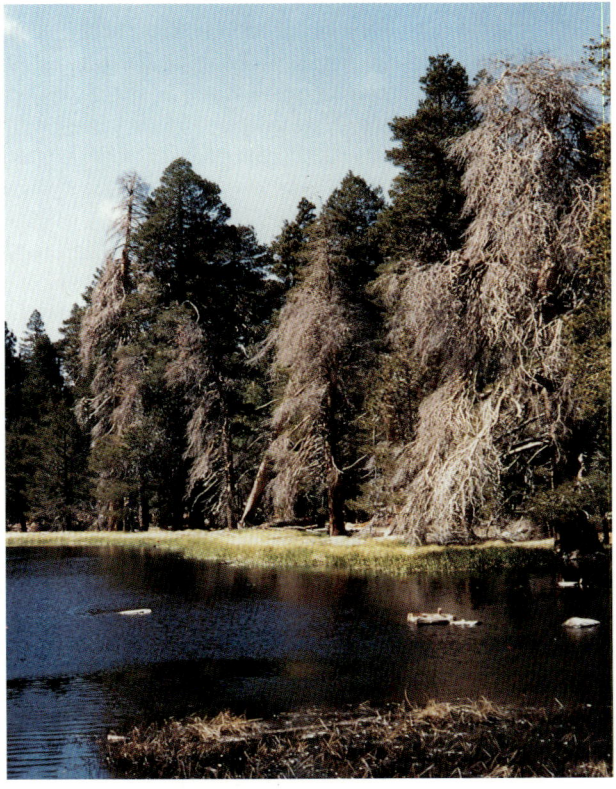

Figure 1-11—
These Jeffrey pines were killed by excess soil moisture when the water table was changed by a new beaver pond.

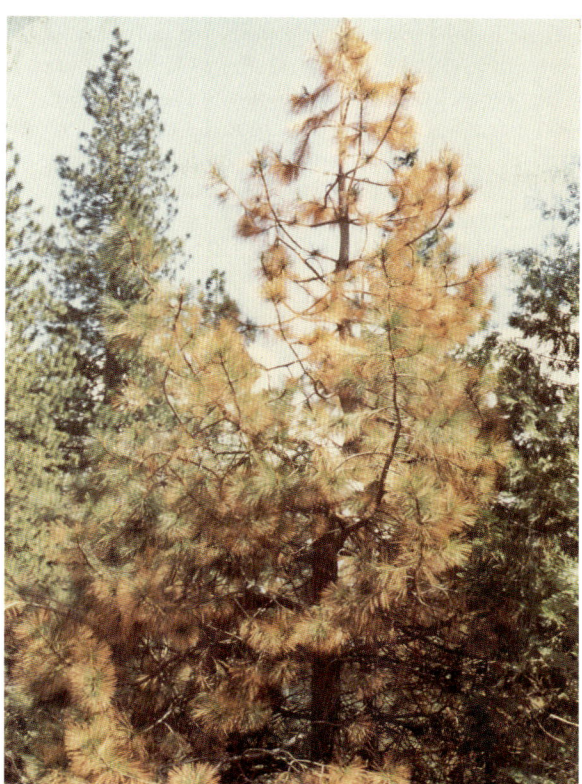

Figure 1-12—*Absorption of chloride salts from deicing compounds applied to highways can cause severe needle necrosis, as seen in this Jeffrey pine.*

established lawns often die. In all cases, damage is caused by the depletion of the oxygen supply to the roots. Damage may range from moderate (greenish yellow or brown foliage throughout the crown) to severe (death of major branches or the entire tree). Excess soil moisture may also encourage "water mold" fungi, which cause serious root rots—particularly in ornamental plantings on former agricultural soils.

There may be some differences in species response to high water table. For example, lodgepole pine may persist longer under these conditions than ponderosa pine.

EXCESS MINERALS

Excess salt

Roadside environment—The uptake of chloride ions by the roots of roadside trees or from direct foliar contact with salt is a common problem wherever sodium chloride and calcium chloride are applied to icy highways in the winter (fig. 1-12). Highway maintenance programs sometimes use borate salts for weed control along roadsides (see Herbicide Toxicity). Many roadside trees are killed by chloride and borate salts. In the Lake Tahoe Basin of California and Nevada, the average distances from the edges of highways to trees showing different salt damage ratings were 41 feet (13 m), no damage; 21 feet (6 m), light damage; 20 feet (6 m), moderate damage; and 15 feet (5 m), severe damage. The final result of salt accumulation in conifer foliage is needle tip dieback. The cause can be confirmed by analysis of leaf tissue and soil for chloride content. The dead tissue is reddish brown and may occupy as little as 1 inch (2 to 3 cm) of the needle tip or as much as the entire needle. The increased salt content of the soil also decreases water uptake by trees, thus inducing an artificial drought.

Coastal environment—Salt damage may be expected in locations along the coast where trees have been planted on landfill, such as marinas. Eventually, the roots of these trees grow down to the salty water table. The damage is characterized by reddish-brown needle tip dieback, yellowing of living needle tissue, and reduced needle length.

Salt damage can also be expected some distance from the beach or oceanfront where salt spray is blown onto trees. After a storm with high winds along the central California coast, only the windward side of trees had brown needles; the damage was observed up to 0.25 mile (0.4 km) from the beach. Occasional storm-related salt injury causes no lasting damage. A common foliar damage to coast redwood has been attributed to salt spray. The "flag" growth form of cypresses and other conifers may result from the combination of wind pressure and constant salt absorption, which together cause death of needles, buds, and twigs (fig. 1-13).

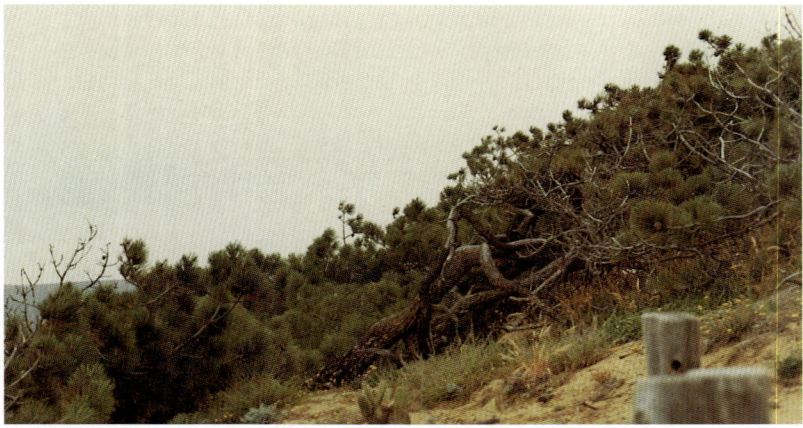

Figure 1-13—*The prostrate forms of Torrey pines growing on the bluffs immediately above the ocean may have resulted from both wind pressure and gradual absorption of windborne salts by foliage.*

Excess fertilizer

Nitrogen compounds in excessive amounts can cause "burning" of needle tips. Christmas tree plantations, nurseries, and other locations where trees receive intensive care are the places where fertilizer burn is usually found. It may also be confused with injury by selective herbicides applied in excess to the soil. Recovery from injury by excess nitrogen may be expected to be more rapid than recovery from herbicide injury.

Sewage effluent

Trees growing near places of habitation may receive sewage water from drainage fields or treatment plants, and some forests have been fertilized with treated sewage effluent. After an initial growth stimulation, trees show symptoms resembling those caused by soil sterilants (such as boron) in the second year; some trees can be expected to die thereafter. Jeffrey pine, sugar pine, and white firs have been killed in the vicinity of leach lines.

Serpentine soils

Soils derived from serpentine, an igneous rock, occupy 1,100 square miles (1770 km^2) in Lake, Napa, Marin, and Sonoma Counties, and in some Mother Lode counties of California, as well as 450 square miles (724 km^2) in the Siskiyou Mountains of Oregon, and 200 square miles (322 km^2) in Washington. The presence of serpentine soils is often signaled by an abrupt change of vegetation type or a reduction of tree stature along a distinct line—the contact between normal and serpentine soils. The serpentine side has the appearance of being severely grazed or burned. In Lake County, a sparse kind of chaparral, including Digger pine, is present on the soils derived from serpentine. When serpentine soils occur in the range of the California pine and mixed conifer types, only Jeffrey pine and incense-cedar can persist.

The exclusion of many species and dwarfing of trees on serpentine soils is attributed to their unique mineral content. The content of exchangeable magnesium is extremely high, whereas content of calcium, potassium, nitrogen, and phosphorus is extremely low. Chromium and nickel content is very high, whereas molybdenum content is often deficient. Poor growth is attributed to nutrient imbalance.

MINERAL DEFICIENCY

Deficiency of the major nutrients—nitrogen, phosphorus, and potassium—might be expected if trees are planted on land formerly used to grow agricultural crops, for example, Christmas tree plantations. Nitrogen deficiency shows as chlorosis of the older needles and stunted growth. Phosphorus deficiency results in a purple discoloration and withering of older foliage. Potassium deficiency causes chlorosis and needle tip dieback of older needles. The symptoms of nutritional deficiency in Monterey pine are well illustrated in color by a publication of the New Zealand Forest Service (Will 1985).

HERBICIDE TOXICITY

Chemical herbicide applications are usually associated with particular land-use situations, including the control of brush around dwellings, on fuelbreaks, and along roadsides, railroad tracks, and powerline rights-of-way. Damage to desirable species at the edge of the control area is usually caused by accidental application or drift of the spray droplets onto foliage and by root absorption of herbicide that falls to the ground when it is applied to surfaces of nearby trees.

The symptoms of herbicide injury to conifers are not as well known as those on herbaceous plants. Some categories of symptoms to expect include twisting of needles and shoots and needle necrosis due to hormone-type herbicides such as 2,4-D, and trichloropyr (Garlon 4) (fig. 1-14); severe stunting caused by glyphosate (Roundup or Accord); chlorosis and necrosis from root-absorbed herbicides of the triazine group (hexazinone [Velpar or Pronone], atrazine, and simizine), or substituted ureas (Linuron); and yellow-white bleaching from aminotrizole (Amitrol).

Conifers usually recover from hormone-type herbicides with little lasting damage. Herbicides that are absorbed by roots on one side of the tree may damage only that foliage supplied by those roots. Root-absorbed herbicides usually cause death or lasting damage in the most severe cases. Sugar pine, incense-cedar, and junipers are particularly sensitive to hexazinone (Velpar or Pronone). Herbicides like simizine, which are used to control weeds selectively in Christmas tree plantations, cause injury to Monterey pines only if soils are sandy.

AIR POLLUTANTS

Particulates

Solid particles such as fly ash, road dust, or dust from cement plants are often harmful to conifers in the immediate vicinity of the source. The particles injure the trees by preventing light from reaching the surface of the needles, thereby reducing photosynthesis. In some cases, the cement dust or fly ash may have toxic components that injure the needle tissue directly. Both effects result in premature defoliation of the tree. Damage can be expected only in the immediate vicinity of the source because all but the smallest particles settle

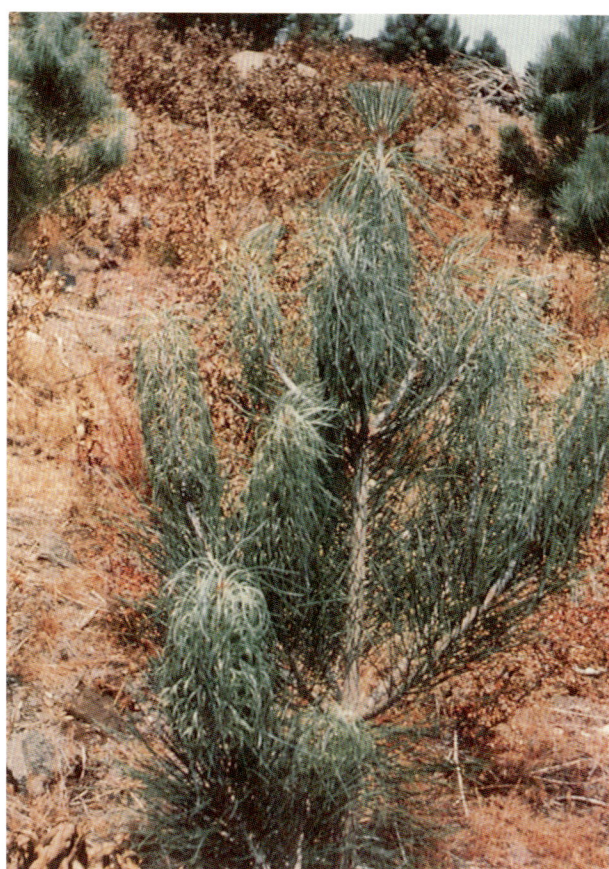

Figure 1-14—
Damage by 2,4-D spray drift occurring after needle elongation caused yellowing and drooping of the old needles of Coulter pine.

out rapidly. Road dust may also inhibit the reproduction of predators of pine leaf scales, thus allowing scale infestations to become more severe.

Gaseous pollutants

Gaseous air pollutants are dispersed over much wider areas than particulate pollutants. Sources may be classified as

1. Point sources—for example, the stack of a power-generating plant or factory.
2. Non-point (area) sources—for example, a metropolitan area, agricultural waste and chemicals, etc.

Topography and local meteorological conditions are important factors that determine the degree to which pollutants concentrate in the atmosphere. These two factors define air basins, which are regions sharing a common air mass and meteorological conditions.

The meteorological conditions most responsible for concentrations of air pollutants include the radiation temperature inversion, which is typical of inland valleys, and the marine temperature inversion, which is found in coastal valleys. The distinctive feature of the temperature inversions is a layer of warm air sandwiched in between a lower layer of cool air near the ground where pollutants concentrate and an upper layer of cool, relatively clean air. This structure prevents the upward dispersion of pollutants. The prevailing windspeed and direction determine the horizontal transport of the pollutants. Low windspeed enhances concentration of pollutants. Both the inland flow of marine air and the daytime upcanyon or upslope flow on sun-heated mountain slopes transport pollutants concentrated beneath the inversion layer to forested areas.

Ozone—The air pollutant most damaging to conifers in California is ozone (O_3). Ozone is the major plant-damaging constituent of photochemical oxidant air pollution (smog). The source of this pollution includes automobiles and various fossil fuel-burning industrial sources. Ozone is not emitted directly from automobiles or smoke stacks but rather is formed by a complex chemical reaction in the atmosphere. Two primary pollutants, nitrogen dioxide and hydrocarbons (from gasoline vapor, organic solvents, etc.), react with sunlight to produce ozone.

Ozone damage is most severe in the mountains of southern California and on the west side of the southern Sierra Nevada. Ponderosa pines showing even moderate to severe injury by ozone are more frequently attacked and killed by bark beetles than healthy trees.

Ozone-damaged trees are typically distributed on mountain slopes and crests that form the border of an air basin (for example, between coastal and desert areas) and downwind (in the predominant summer direction) from heavily populated areas. Trees are damaged as far as 80 miles (129 km) east of the Los Angeles metropolitan area. The distribution of affected trees at a particular site is quite random, indicating that there is a high degree of genetic variability in sensitivity within the species.

Ponderosa and Jeffrey pines are the first species to show injury, and the amount of injury under field conditions to these pines can be identified with five descriptive categories.

1. *None*—four or more annual needle whorls are retained, with no evidence of yellow or chlorotic mottle on any needles.
2. *Possible injury*—four or more annual needle whorls are retained but oldest whorl(s) display distinct chlorotic needle mottle (fig. 1-15) and sometimes may be easily pulled from the stem.
3. *Slight injury*—three or four annual needle whorls are retained, with distinct chlorotic mottle on older needle whorls accompanied by premature needle abscission of oldest needles. The length

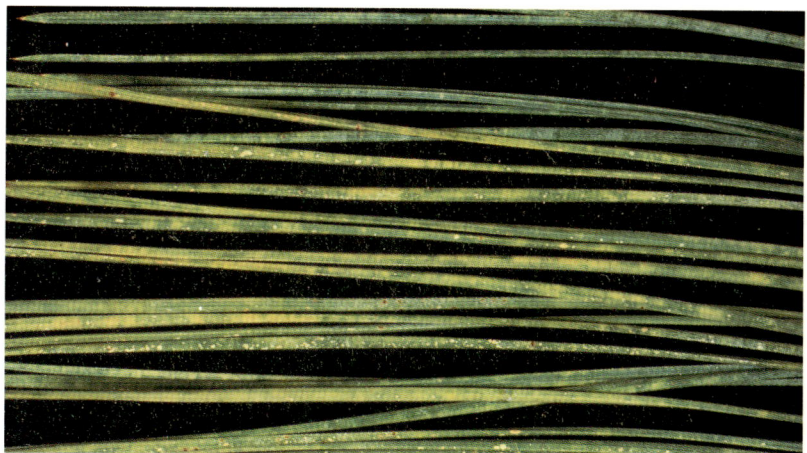

Figure 1-15—*Ponderosa pine needles show the chlorotic mottle symptom that is the principal diagnostic feature of ozone injury to pines. Mottle advances from needle tip to base and is always more intense on older needle whorls.*

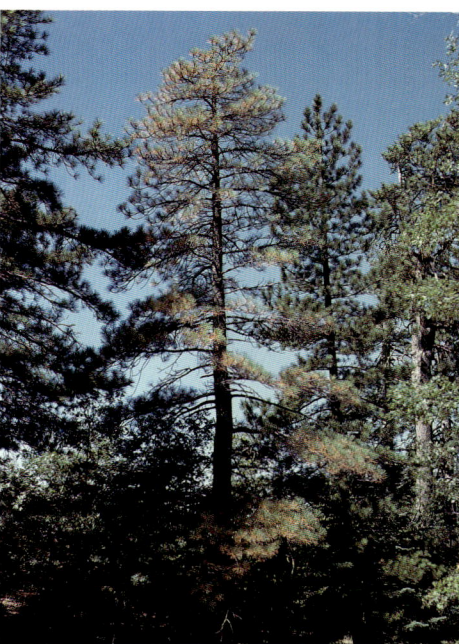

Figure 1-16—*During winter, only shortened current-year needles remain on this ponderosa pine severely damaged by ozone.*

of recent annual shoot growth may be reduced. Lowest branches show the most defoliation.
4. *Moderate injury*—two to three annual whorls are retained, with intensification of other symptoms described under "slight injury."
5. *Severe injury*—one or two annual needle whorls are retained in late summer, both with shortened yellow mottled needles with or without tip necrosis of the current and 1-year-old needles (fig. 1-16). Older needles fall easily from the stem. Chronic

suppression of shoot growth is evident. Apical dominance is often diminished, resulting in a flat-topped crown. Lower and mid-crown branches are dead (fig. 1-16). Ozone injury to white fir develops according to the same sequence of events.

In fumigation trials with 1- to 3-year-old seedlings, the following species of western conifers were ranked in the order of decreasing ozone sensitivity: ponderosa pine, Jeffrey pine, white fir, Coulter pine, red fir, knobcone pine, incense-cedar, bigcone Douglas-fir, and sugar pine. Until recently, Monterey pines in Christmas tree plantations in southern California showed ozone injury consistently (fig. 1-17). The problems have diminished because vegetative propagation of ozone-tolerant individuals to provide replanting stock has been practiced on a wide scale.

Sulfur dioxide—Sulfur dioxide can be a chronic problem in areas where sulfur-containing coal and oil are burned or where smelters process sulfide ores of copper, zinc, lead, and iron. On conifer needles, sulfur dioxide causes a reddish-brown discoloration that often does not cover the entire needle but occurs in bands beginning at the needle tip. Middle-aged and older needle whorls are injured first, and branches die progressively from the bottom of the tree to the top. Damage can occur anytime—even during mild winter weather.

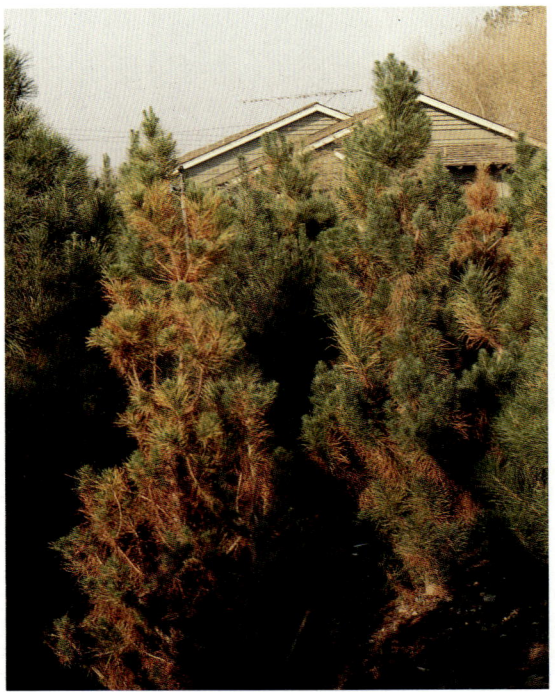

Figure 1-17—
In densely planted Monterey pine Christmas tree plantations, ozone damage is found in all degrees.

Less severe doses cause a chlorosis and premature abscission of older needles. Winter injury and drought symptoms usually cause a brown discoloration of the entire needle but not as reddish as that of sulfur dioxide injury; symptoms appear in spring or late summer, respectively. Drought affects current-year's needles and the upper crown first; winter injury involves older needles as well and is present throughout the crown.

The order of decreasing sulfur dioxide susceptibility of selected western conifers studied is grand fir, subalpine fir, western redcedar, western hemlock, Douglas-fir, western white pine, ponderosa pine, lodgepole pine, western larch, Engelmann spruce, western juniper, and Pacific yew.

Hydrogen fluoride—Fluoride damage to western conifer species was a chronic problem in the vicinity of Spokane, WA, during the 1950's and more recently at Columbia Falls, MT. Hydrogen fluoride is emitted from aluminum ore reduction plants, phosphate fertilizer plants, brick kilns, and glassworks.

The current-year's needles of conifers are the most sensitive to fluoride. Needle tip dieback begins while new needles are elongating in the spring, but the same needles become relatively resistant to further damage later in the season. Needle tips first become chlorotic and then turn brown. The needle tip dieback on older needles does not represent new injury but mainly injury that developed during elongation; these injured needles are usually shed. Foliar analysis for fluoride content is an excellent diagnostic method for confirming the cause if done by a laboratory with adequate experience. Sensitive species include ponderosa pine, western larch, lodgepole pine, and Douglas-fir. Grand fir, blue spruce, and white spruce are less susceptible, whereas arborvitae and juniper are tolerant.

FIRE

Conifers are most susceptible to fire damage early in the growing season when stems and shoots are actively growing. The factors that determine tree survival after fire are the amount of foliage, bud and twig, and bark and cambium killed. Extensive amounts of foliage may be killed without much damage to buds and twigs (fig. 1-18). A tree that overwinters with no live needles may survive unless high temperatures have killed the cambium tissue of the main stem. The early evaluation of fire damage and survivability of ponderosa pine is aided by several key observations: twigs with needles remaining and bent in the direction of the run of the fire are almost always dead; twigs having needles with green bases are likely to be alive. After a few months, needles will fall from living twigs, because an abscission layer is formed, but will remain on dead branches. Other important

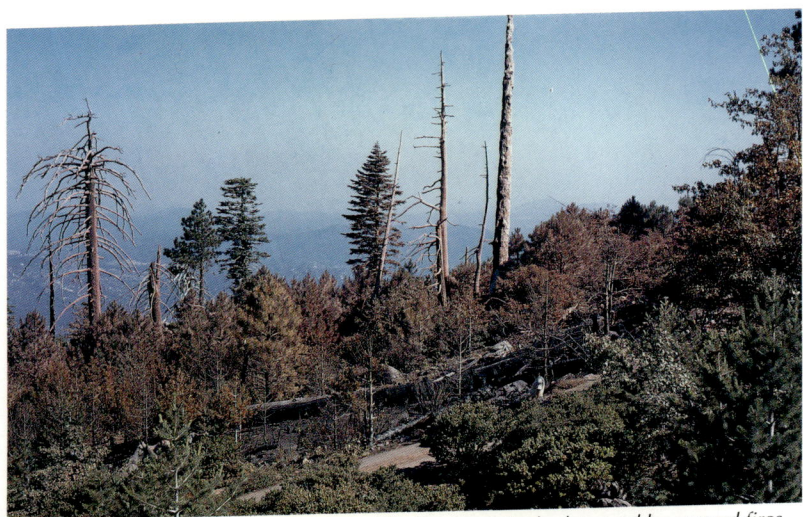

Figure 1-18—Sapling pines are usually killed or extensively damaged by ground fires. Older trees with thicker bark may survive extensive charring of the bark and scorch of needles in the lower crown.

predictors of survival are height of crown scorch and depth of bark char.

Several years after the fire, bark on surviving thin-bark species will commonly scale off. Thicker bark has greater insulating capacity to protect the cambium from injury. Bark thickness varies from species to species and even within a species. The order of decreasing bark thickness, and thus decreasing fire resistance, of some selected western conifers is giant sequoia, redwood, ponderosa pine, Douglas-fir, sugar pine, white pine, California red fir, white fir, grand fir, lodgepole pine, and western redcedar. Other factors that decrease fire sensitivity are deep rooting habit, low amounts of resin in old bark, first branches high above the ground, and open, less-dense branch habit.

Cambium injury is ordinarily heaviest on the lee side of the tree with respect to the direction of run of the fire and on the uphill side of trees located on slopes. Killed patches of cambium are widest just above the ground and taper upward; however, charred heartwood is usually still present as confirming evidence. Heat injury to cambium without extensive charring may eventually result in bark scaling even on species with thick bark (fig. 1-19).

LIGHTNING

The most common evidence of lightning injury to taller trees is a narrow furrow in which the bark and a thin layer of wood are

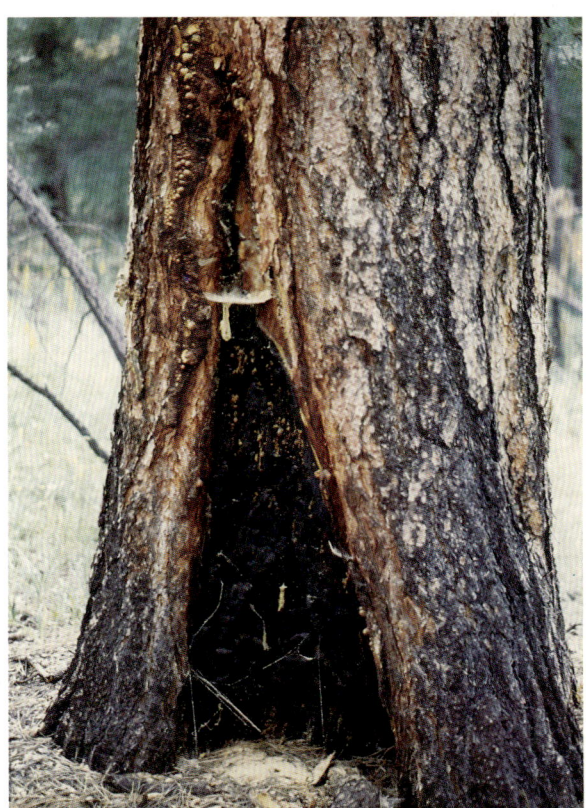

Figure 1-19—
Charred wood remains as healing of fire damage to the lower bole of this ponderosa pine stem proceeds.

damaged. The furrow extends spirally around the trunk from the top of the bole to the butt (fig. 1-20). The tree top may be killed immediately; bark beetles often invade the tree. The generally sharp-edged furrow caused by lightning is easily distinguished from the ribs or cracks resulting from freezing or drought. Some trees, particularly white fir, are completely shattered. Either the top is broken or a large section of the lower bole "explodes" (fig. 1-21). Occasionally small circular groups of conifers may be killed by a diffuse electrical discharge without showing any outward signs of mechanical injury except for a foliage scorch. Some trees struck by lightning, although damaged, survive.

SNOW, ICE, AND MECHANICAL FACTORS

Snow and ice

Heavy snow accumulations often bend or break the stems of younger conifers (fig. 1-22). Typical injuries include a longitudinal split on the lower stem, a stem fracture between base and breast

Figure 1-20—
Lightning injury is typically indicated by a narrow strip of bark removed in a spiral course down the bole.

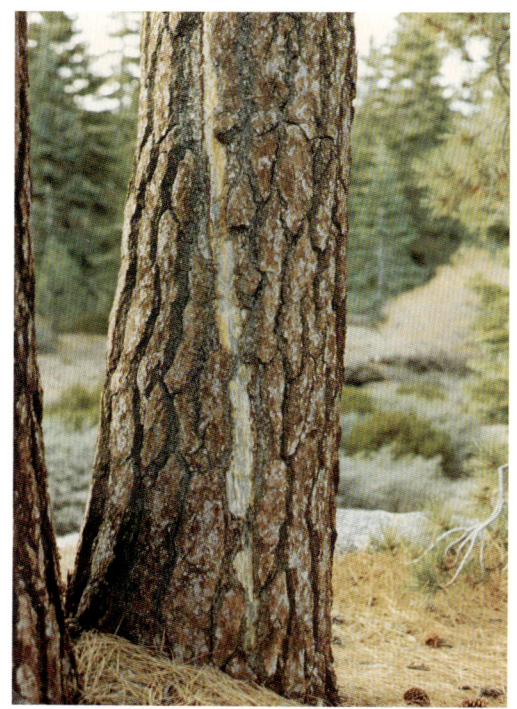

Figure 1-21—
Lightning damage to white fir is often very destructive. This fir essentially exploded on being struck.

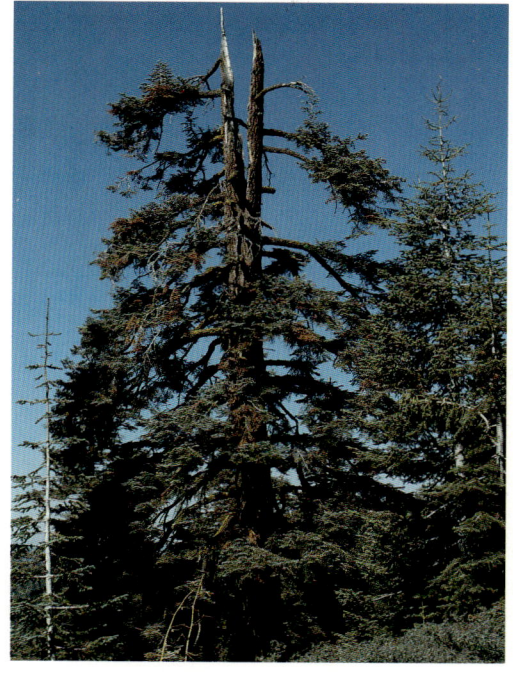

height, or even uprooting. Unbroken, severely bent stems straighten after a few years, but snow bending can significantly reduce height growth the year after injury. Trees in densely stocked stands are more susceptible to damage than trees in the seedling and sapling stage growing in open areas. Small trees may be broken by a dense, heavy snow load falling from an adjacent dominant tree.

Additional damages may result from movement of the snowpack. Changes in crystalline structure cause a plastic deformation of the snowpack that is manifested by vertical settlement, even on gentle slopes. Vertical settlement will tear branches away from the stem. Seedlings and saplings are the most affected. In addition, on steep slopes, creep of the snowpack results from a differential movement in which upper layers move more than lower layers. The entire snowpack (all layers) may glide uniformly downslope at the soil-snow interface. Creep and glide result in permanent stem deformities, including butt or stem sweep (curvature immediately above the ground level) and stem failure.

Rime ice frequently accumulates on ponderosa pine and other dominant conifers along exposed ridgetops. The weight of this ice breaks the tops as well as smaller branches throughout the crown. Larger affected trees may develop broad, flat-topped crowns, whereas boles of pole-sized trees have curves and distortions of the bole

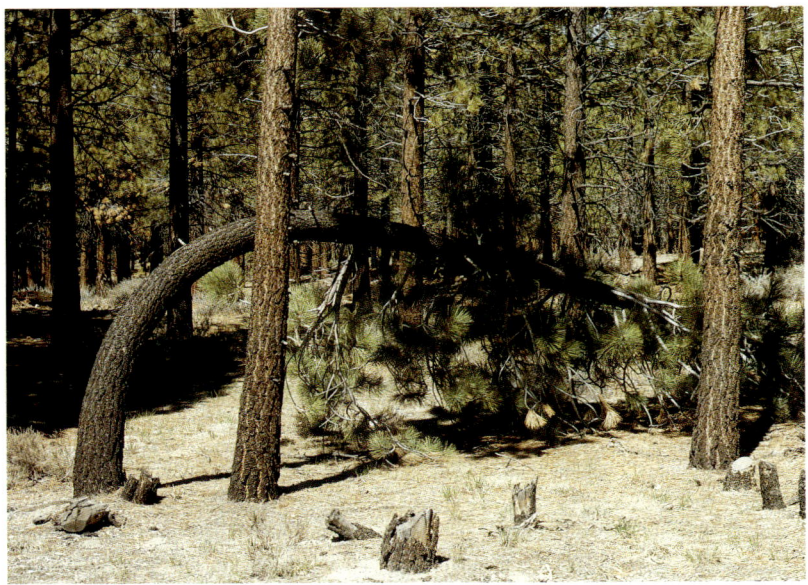

Figure 1-22—*Snow loading causes small trees to remain prostrate temporarily. They usually regain an erect position after several growing seasons unless snow loading occurs repeatedly, as with this Jeffrey pine growing within range of the snow plume of rotary snow plows.*

resulting from lateral branches taking over as terminal leaders.

In areas where rotary snow plows are used, for example, along the Trans-Sierra highways in California, damage to and removal of needles, twigs, and branches are common. The repeated impact of the snow plume of rotary plows and the blast of wind-driven ice particles can result in defoliation of the upper crown above the snowpack (fig. 1-23).

At higher elevations where deep snow is persistent, the freezing and thawing in the top layer produce large ice crystals on the surface. High winds drive these crystals against the bark, and the wood may be exposed in a 2- to 3-foot-long (0.6 to 0.9 m) section on one side of the stem. This injury appears at heights up to 20 feet (6 m) above the ground, depending on snow depth.

Hail

Hail storms cause defoliation, bud injury, and bruising or lesions on the upper side of needles, stems, and young cones. New growth is most susceptible to damage. The worst bruising occurs on upper

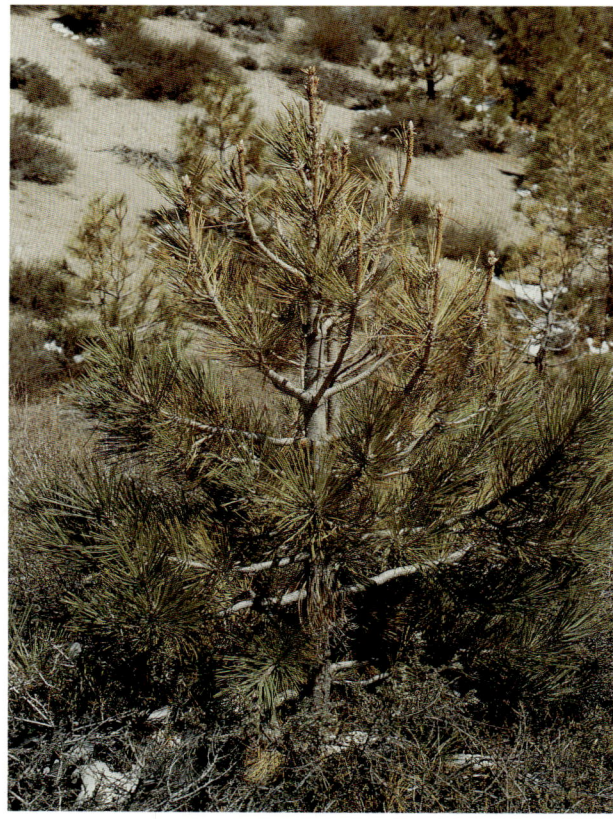

Figure 1-23—
Frequent blasts of wind-driven snow caused extensive defoliation of the upper crowns of this Jeffrey pine sapling. The lower portion of the crown was buried in the snow and was protected from injury.

branches and on the windward sides of trees. Immediately after a storm, many green needles and small shoots can be seen on the ground. Several years after a hailstorm, the most obvious evidence is dead tops and one-sided crowns. Damage is sometimes quite localized in the forest. The species most severely damaged by hail is Douglas-fir; white fir, incense-cedar, sugar pine, and ponderosa pine receive less injury.

Wind

Topography and timber cutting practices are important factors that determine the extent of windthrow. Damage is usually heavy on ridgetops and upper slopes, but downslope winds can cause extensive damage. Winds at 40 to 50 miles (64 to 80 km) per hour streamline or flow with the contour of the slope on the lee side, especially where the mountain barrier is at right angles to the wind. In the most severe situation, a clear-cut area on the windward side of the slope offers no barrier to the wind blowing into a timbered area on the lee side of the slope. As a result, winds blow with greater force along the contour of the lee slope than elsewhere, and windthrow is more frequent.

Other associated factors that favor windthrow, in decreasing order of importance, are snow load; root and butt rot, particularly where roots on the leeward side fail under compression; shallow soils; and wet, poorly drained soils. The tree may also break at any point along the main stem, for example, at rust cankers, a beaver girdle, or where the bole is hollowed by fire. Trees with a high taper (low values of height per diameter at breast height) are more wind-stable than those of the same height and crown type but of low taper. Swellings may develop at places where the stem was cracked by wind but failed to break.

Some dominant trees that undergo constant wind rock tend to develop much sturdier root systems than those in the interior of a stand. It is common for individual trees left standing in a heavily cutover area to be windthrown within the first 2 years after the cut. Windthrown trees create longer term problems; for example, weakened trees are susceptible to bark beetle attack, and heavy loading of large-diameter fuel can increase damage by fire. Extensive windthrow has been reported frequently in the Pacific Northwest and in the Sierra Nevada.

HUMAN ACTIVITIES

Construction activities can damage trees in several ways. Stems can be debarked by equipment. Digging and earth-moving activities can sever large portions of the root system, and the weight of equip-

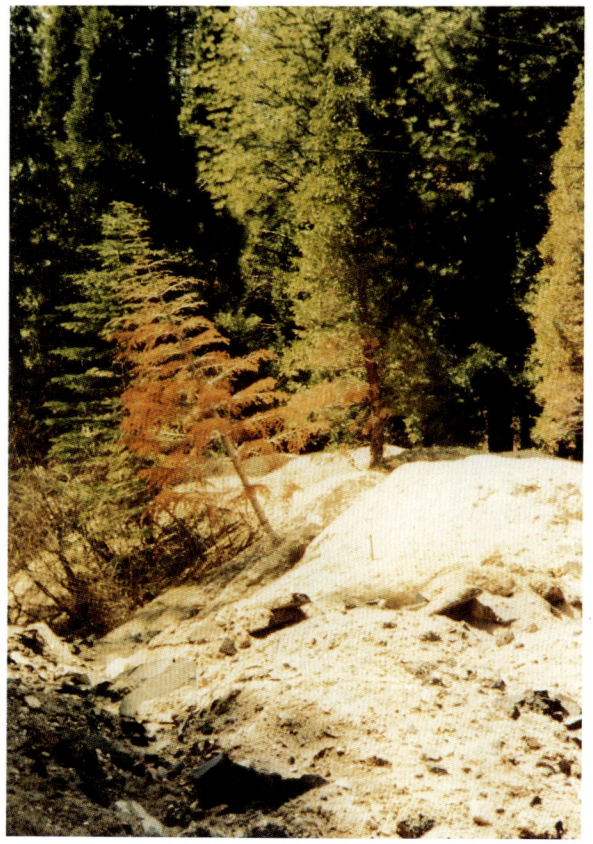

Figure 1-24— *Incense-cedar killed by the anaerobic conditions induced when the dirt, rocks, and chunks of asphalt were dumped over the roots.*

ment can cause soil compaction. Stressed trees are more susceptible to windthrow, stem decay, and bark beetle attack. Root systems buried by earth fill or asphalt pavement or silt washed downhill from construction sites have diminished oxygen supply and the tree may die in a single season (fig. 1-24).

The growth rates of larger conifers observed in public campgrounds throughout California have not revealed any changes over a 30-year period that could be directly related to recreational use. Young conifers, however, were susceptible to damage in recreation areas, particularly from vandalism. No seedlings of the smallest size category were observed at any of several recreation sites, and larger seedlings, saplings, and poles had generally decreased in number.

Timber harvesting practices can have an important effect on the condition and survival of remaining trees. In a comparison of bole damage resulting from different cutting methods in Douglas-fir, 22 percent of remaining trees were damaged by overstory removal, 12 percent by selection, and 6 percent by understory removal.

SELECTED REFERENCES

Anonymous. 1967. Forest pest conditions in California—1967. Sacramento, CA: California Forest Pest Action Council, California Division of Forestry. 20 p.

Anonymous. 1968. Forest pest conditions in California—1968. Sacramento, CA: California Forest Pest Action Council, California Division of Forestry. 16 p.

Benson, Robert E. 1980. Damage from logging and prescribed burning in partially cut Douglas-fir stands. Res. Note INT-294. Ogden, UT: U.S. Department of Agriculture, Forest Service, Intermountain Forest and Range Experiment Station. 6 p.

Bentley, Jay R.; Blakeman, D.A.; Cooper, S.B. 1971. Recovery of young ponderosa pines damaged by herbicide spraying. Res. Note PSW-252. Berkeley, CA: U.S. Department of Agriculture, Forest Service, Pacific Southwest Forest and Range Experiment Station. 7 p.

Brown, A.A.; Davis, K.P. 1973. Forest fire: control and use. 2d. ed. New York: McGraw-Hill. 686 p.

Gordon, Donald T. 1973. Damage from wind and other causes in mixed white-red fir stands adjacent to clearcuttings. Res. Pap. PSW-90. Berkeley, CA: U.S. Department of Agriculture, Forest Service, Pacific Southwest Forest and Range Experiment Station. 22 p.

Grier, Charles C. 1988. Foliage loss due to snow, wind, and winter drying damage: its effects on leaf biomass of some western conifer forests. Canadian Journal of Forest Research 18:1097–1102.

Hadley, J.L.; Smith, W.K. 1983. Influence of wind exposure on needle desiccation and mortality for timberline conifers in Wyoming, U.S.A. Arctic and Alpine Research 15:127–135.

Jacobson, Jay S.; Hill, Clyde A., eds. 1970. Recognition of air pollution injury to vegetation: a pictorial atlas. Pittsburgh, PA: Air Pollution Control Association. 102 p.

Kangur, R. 1973. Snow damage to young mixed forests of western hemlock and Douglas-fir. Res. Pap. 21. Corvallis: Oregon State University, Forest Research Laboratory, School of Forestry. 11 p.

Kruckeberg, A.R. 1984. California serpentines: flora, vegetation, geology, soils, and management problems. Berkeley: University of California Press. 180 p.

Larsen, J.B. 1981. Geographic variation in winter drought resistance of Douglas-fir (*Pseudotsuga menziesii* Mirb. Franco). Silvae Genetica 30:4–5.

Leaphart, Charles D.; Hungerford, R.D.; Johnson, H.E. 1972. Stem deformities in young trees caused by snowpack and its movement. Res. Note INT-158. Ogden, UT: U.S. Department of Agriculture, Forest Service, Intermountain Forest and Range Experiment Station. 10 p.

Leaphart, Charles D.; Stage, Albert R. 1971. Climate: a factor in the origin of pole blight disease of *Pinus monticola* Dougl. Ecology 52(2):229–239.

Lund-Huie, K.; Bayer, D.E. 1968. Absorption, translocation, and metabolism of 3-amino-1,2,3-triazole in *Pinus ponderosa* and *Abies concolor*. Physiologia Plantarum 21:196–212.

Magill, Arthur W. 1970. Five California campgrounds...conditions improve after 5 years recreational use. Res. Pap. PSW-62. Berkeley, CA: U.S. Department of Agriculture, Forest Service, Pacific Southwest Forest and Range Experiment Station. 18 p.

Miller, Douglas R. 1970. In: Key and guides to the damaging forest pests of California. San Francisco: U.S. Department of Agriculture, Forest Service, Pacific Southwest Region. (unpublished manuscript).

Miller, Paul R.; Millecan, Arthur A. 1971. Extent of oxidant air pollution damage to some pines and other conifers in California. Plant Disease Reporter 55(6): 555–559.

Miller, P.R.; Longbotham, G.J.; Longbotham, C.R. 1983. Sensitivity of selected western conifers to ozone. Plant Disease 67:1113–1115.

Oliver, William W. 1970. Snow bending of sugar pine and ponderosa pine seedlings—injury not permanent. Res. Note PSW-225. Berkeley, CA: U.S. Department of Agriculture, Forest Service, Pacific Southwest Forest and Range Experiment Station. 3 p.

Perry, T.O.; Baldwin, G.W. 1966. Winter breakdown of the photosynthetic apparatus of evergreen species. Forest Science 12:298–300.

Peterson, David L.; Arbaugh, Michael J. 1989. Estimating postfire survival of Douglas-fir in the Cascade Range. Canadian Journal of Forest Research 19:530–533.

Petty, J.A.; Swain, C. 1985. Factors influencing stem breakage of conifers in high winds. Forestry 58:75–84.

Scharpf, Robert F.; Srago, Michael. 1974. Conifer damage and death associated with the use of highway deicing salt in the Lake Tahoe Basin of California and Nevada. Forest Pest Control Tech. Rep. 1. San Francisco: U.S. Department of Agriculture, Forest Service, California Region. 16 p.

Scheffer, Theodore C.; Hedgecock, George G. 1955. Injury to Northwestern forest trees by sulfur dioxide from smelters. Tech. Bull. 1117. Washington, DC: U.S. Department of Agriculture. 49 p.

Stewart, Dennis; Treshow, Michael; Harner, Francis M. 1973. Pathological anatomy of conifer needle necrosis. Canadian Journal of Botany 51(5):983–988.

Wagener, Willis W. 1949. Top dying of conifers from sudden cold. Journal of Forestry 47:49–53.

Wagener, Willis W. 1960. A comment on cold susceptibility of ponderosa and Jeffrey pines. Madrono 15:217–219.

Wagener, Willis W. 1961. Guidelines for estimating the survival of fire damaged trees in California. Misc. Pap. 60. Berkeley, CA: U.S. Department of Agriculture, Forest Service, Pacific Southwest Forest and Range Experiment Station. 11 p.

Walker, R.B. 1954. Ecology of serpentine soils: II. factors affecting plant growth on serpentine soils. Ecology 35:259–266.

Westing, Arthur H. 1969. Symposium on soil and water pollution damage to plants—plants and salt in the roadside environment. Phytopathology 59:1174–1191.

Will, Graham. 1985. Nutrient deficiencies and fertilizer use in New Zealand exotic forests. Bull. No. 97. Rotorua, New Zealand: New Zealand Forest Service, Forest Research Institute. 55 p.

CHAPTER 2   Needle Diseases

Richard S. Smith, Jr. and Robert F. Scharpf

Principal Plant Pathologist, Forest Insect and Disease Research Staff, Forest Service, U.S. Department of Agriculture, Washington, DC, formerly with the Pacific Southwest Forest and Range Experiment Station and the Pacific Southwest Region
Research Scientist Emeritus; formerly Project Leader, Disease Research and Principal Plant Pathologist, Pacific Southwest Research Station, Forest Service, U.S. Department of Agriculture, Albany, CA.

INTRODUCTION

Most conifers depend upon a 2- to 11-year complement of needles for maximum growth and development. When a large portion of these needles die, they are not replaced—and the growth of the tree is reduced. Complete defoliation is usually fatal.

Many agents are responsible for needle death. Older needles die naturally and are cast after a certain number of years on the tree. Some insects such as mites, scale, and aphids may kill needles. Abiotic factors, such as air pollution, herbicide sprays, salt injury, over-fertilization, high temperature, drought, and winter injury (red belt), kill needles or parts of them. Rust fungi may also cause needle diseases (chapter 4). Root diseases (chapter 6) may cause needles to yellow and die prematurely.

This chapter concerns needle diseases caused by fungi other than the rust fungi. Most of these diseases can be identified by the characteristic fruiting bodies of the causal fungi that are found on the dead needles or dead portions of partially killed needles. These fungi often have life cycles that are timed with the growth and development of the host and may require 1, 2, or more years to complete.

Sporulation, spread, and infection by these fungi are frequently restricted to a specific season, such as spring, summer, or fall, and successful infection depends on whether conditions are favorable at the time. For example, in some needlecasts, infection is frequently restricted to the newly developing needles, and sporulation is timed to coincide in spring with needle development. These rather rigid requirements for infection in some species result in only an occasional year of heavy infection on 1 year's set of needles. Consequently, the host is usually not completely defoliated and is not killed, but its growth rate may be reduced.

NEEDLE DISEASES COMMON TO SEVERAL GENERA

Brown Felt Blight
Herpotrichia juniperi
Herpotrichia coulteri

Hosts—Brown felt blight is a foliage disease of conifers caused by two similar fungi, *Herpotrichia juniperi* and *H. coulteri*. In North America, *H. coulteri* attacks the foliage of pines only, whereas *H. juniperi* attacks conifers other than pines. Macroscopically, these two fungi are indistinguishable; their effects on the hosts are identical; and their life cycles are quite similar. Traditionally, these two fungi have been treated the same way. They are commonly but erroneously referred to as "snow mold."

Distribution and damage—Brown felt blight is distributed worldwide and is generally found throughout the coniferous forests of North America. The two fungi usually are found only at the higher elevations of mountainous regions, where enough snow falls to meet the unique requirements of these fungi.

The disease develops only under cover of snow; therefore, its attacks are limited to smaller trees and the lower branches of larger trees that are buried under snow in the winter. These fungi envelop twigs and needles in a dark-brown, felt-like growth. Needles within the felt are infected and killed. This disease may, on occasion, kill seedlings and saplings that are covered by snow, but it has little effect on trees once they reach pole size. The damage done in the forest is minimal, but at times it has been a serious problem in snow-covered forest nurseries.

Disease cycle—Infection of the host branch occurs under the snow during winter. The exact source of infection is unknown, but it has been suggested that it originates from infested litter on the forest floor. Under cover of snow, the fungus envelops the branch in a gray mycelium. After snowmelt and exposure, the fungus felt stops growing and turns a dark brown. The following summer the mycelium remains inactive. The second winter, fruiting bodies (perithecia) develop on the felt under the snow. The fruiting bodies remain immature while the infected twig is on the tree, but ripen in late summer on the fallen twigs. Their role in the infection cycle is uncertain.

Field identification—This disease is easily identified in the field by the dense, dark brown mat of mycelium that envelops the needles and twigs (fig. 2-1). Small, black, spherical fruiting bodies can be seen on the second-year mycelial mats.

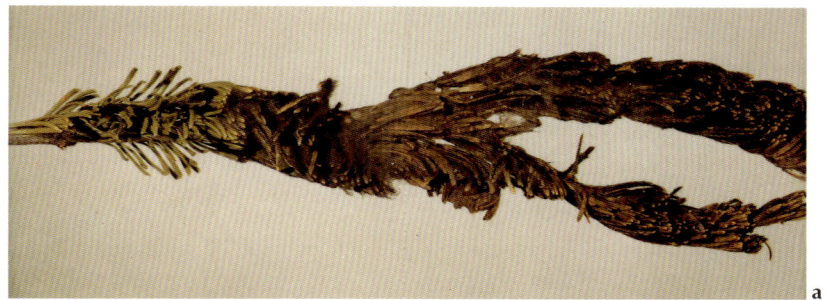
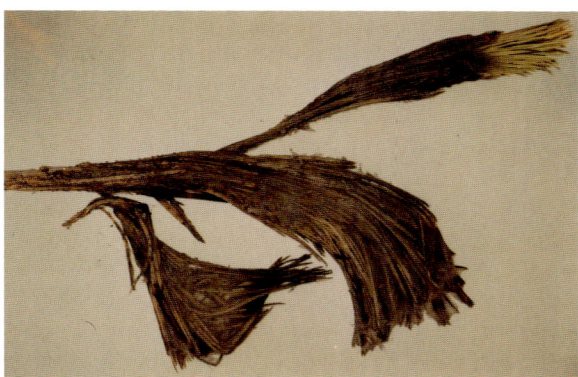

Figure 2-1—The brown fungus mat of brown felt blight covering the ends of branches of a California red fir (**a**) and a sugar pine (**b**).

SPRUCE NEEDLE DISEASES

Lophodermium crassum
Lophodermium piceae

Two minor needle pathogens of spruce are found in the western United States. *Lophodermium crassum* has been reported on Brewer spruce in Siskiyou County, CA. *Lophodermium piceae* has been found on Sitka and Engelmann spruces.

In *L. piceae*, the black, elliptical fruiting bodies occur in longitudinal rows on either side of the middle ridge of the outer faces of the needles. The areas occupied by one or a group of fruiting bodies are separated from one another by heavy black lines extending through the needle and along which the needle readily breaks. *L. crassum* is very similar. These two species can be distinguished only by a cross-sectional view of the fruiting bodies. *L. piceae* is intraepidermal; *L. crassum* is subepidermal.

NEEDLE DISEASES OF LARCH

Larch Needle Blight
Hypodermella laricis
Larch Needle Cast
Meria laricis

Hosts—*Hypodermella laricis* and *Meria laricis* are found on western larch.

Distribution and damage—Both larch needle blight (caused by *Hypodermella laricis*) and larch needle cast (caused by *Meria laricis*) appear sporadically in Oregon, Washington, Idaho, Montana, and British Columbia. Larch in forest stands generally do not experience serious damage from these diseases, even though the diseases may appear to be causing spectacular amounts of foliage mortality. Larch needle cast can kill nursery seedlings, however.

Disease cycle—*Hypodermella laricis* overwinters in dead needles on the host. *Meria laricis* overwinters in dead needles on the host or on the ground. Both fungi produce spores in early spring when larches break bud. Spores are disseminated by wind or rain splash and infect newly emerging needles. Moist conditions favor infection. Mature needles are immune to *Hypodermella laricis*. *Meria laricis* may continue to infect needles through the summer if moisture conditions are favorable.

Field identification—Both pathogens cause larch foliage to turn reddish brown (fig. 2-2). Damage caused by *Hypodermella laricis* first appears in June. Needles are discolored over their entire length, and usually all needles on a spur are affected. Small, black fruiting bodies (hysterothecia) are formed on the dead needles. Dead needles usually remain on the tree for a year before they fall off. Damage by *Meria laricis* appears slightly earlier in the year, often in May. Needle discoloration usually involves only part of the individual infected needle, often appearing first at the tips and spreading downward. Not all needles on each individual spur are affected. Needles in the lower portions of tree crowns are affected first. Fruiting occurs through stomatal openings on the underside of needles and is difficult to detect without special staining techniques. Infected needles usually fall from the tree earlier than normal.

NEEDLE DISEASES OF CYPRESS, JUNIPER, AND CEDAR

Lophodermium juniperi

In the western United States, *Lophodermium juniperi* occurs on junipers and incense-cedar. There is little indication that it is parasitic. The fungus forms small, shiny, black elliptical fruiting bodies on the leaves of the host. It is quite common on many ornamental junipers in city plantings.

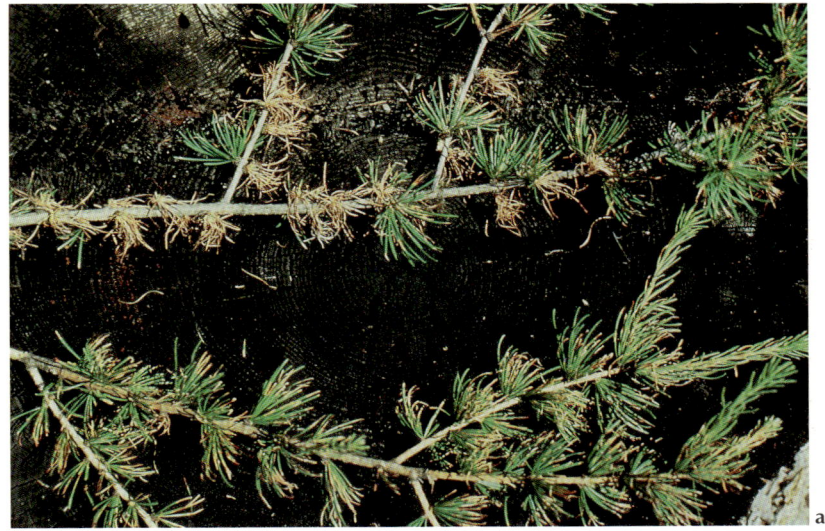

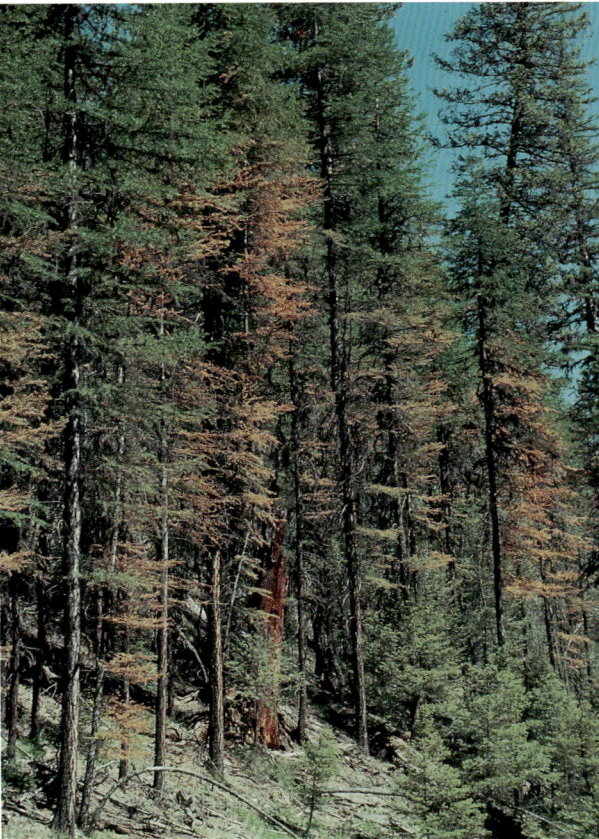

Figure 2-2—
Larch needle blight caused by Hypodermella laricis (**top**) *and larch needle cast caused by* Meria laricis (**bottom**) *infect and kill needles of western larch (**a**). Western larch can suffer widespread killing of foliage by* Meria laricis (**b**).

Cedar Leaf Blight
Didymascella thujina

Cedar leaf blight is a needle disease of the cedars and incense-cedar caused by *Didymascella thujina*. Native to North America and introduced into Europe, this disease is severest on seedlings and young saplings and on the lower branches of older trees growing in dense stands. The foliage is attacked and in severe cases appears as if scorched by fire. In spring, circular to elliptical olive-brown to black fruiting bodies are formed in the upper surfaces of infected leaves (fig. 2-3). These are exposed by the rupture of the covering host epidermis. In late autumn, many young infected twigs drop off. On the remaining leaves, the presence of the disease is easily recognized

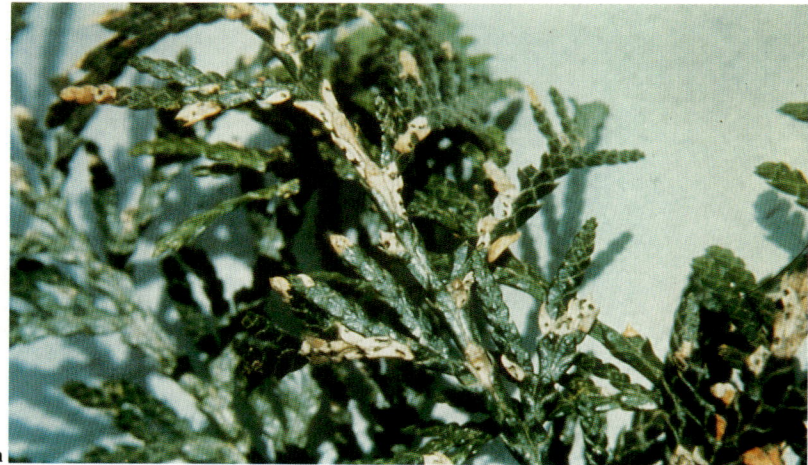

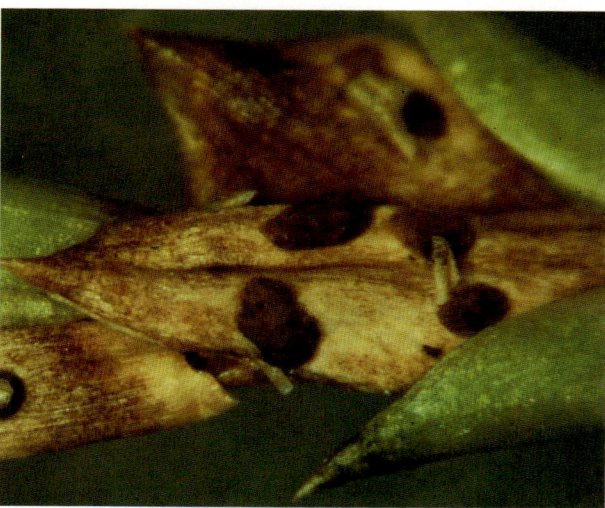

Figure 2-3—*Cedar leaf blight caused by* Didymascella thujina *infects and kills the scale-like needles of western redcedar (**a**). Conspicuous, black fruiting bodies develop on the upper surface of dead infected needles (**b**).*

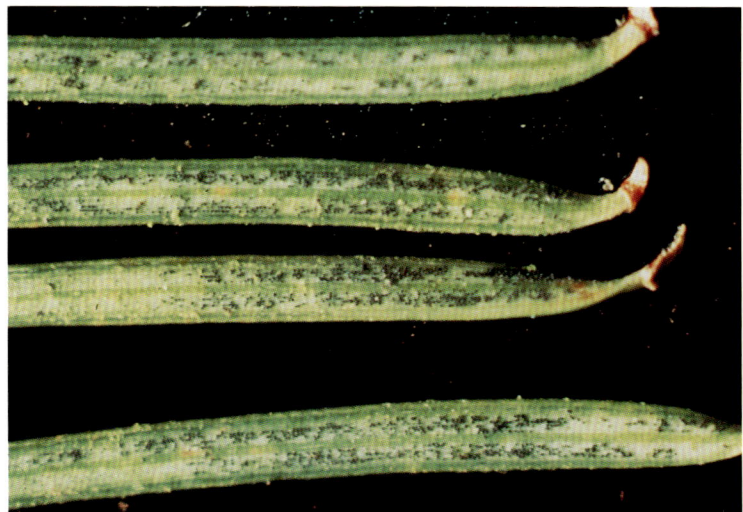

Figure 2-4—*The small, black fruiting bodies of the Swiss needle cast fungus* Phaeocryptopus gaumanni *protrude from the stomata on the underside of an infected Douglas-fir needle.*

by the deep pits that remain in the leaves after the fruiting bodies drop out. The disease is of little or no economic importance in native stands in the western United States but has caused problems on incense-cedar growing in nurseries.

DOUGLAS-FIR NEEDLE DISEASES

Swiss Needle Cast
Phaeocryptopus gaumanni

Swiss needle cast, caused by the fungus *Phaeocryptopus gaumanni,* damages Douglas-fir in Asia, Europe, and parts of North America. It has been most damaging in Switzerland and in neighboring countries where it was first found. Along the Pacific Coast, where both the host and fungus are native, the disease causes little or no damage except on sites where the host is not well adapted, especially Christmas tree plantations. The fungus attacks the host's needles, causing them to yellow, brown, and finally drop. Needle loss is most noticeable in the lower part of the crown. The infected current-year's needles die and are cast over a 1- to 3-year period. No symptoms or signs of infection appear the first year after infection. Only needles 2 years or older show such signs. The small fruiting bodies push their way through the stomata in fall and winter and mature in the spring. Spores are released in May and June. The numerous, small, black spherical fruiting bodies appear as soot-like streaks on the undersurface of the needle along each side of the mid-rib (fig. 2-4).

Douglas-Fir Needle Casts
Rhabdocline pseudotsugae
Rhabdocline weirii

Hosts—The two hosts of Douglas-fir needle cast are Douglas-fir and bigcone Douglas-fir.

Distribution and damage—Douglas-fir needle cast, the single-most important needle disease of Douglas-fir, is caused by two subspecies of *Rhabdocline pseudotsugae* and three subspecies of *R. weirii*. Inasmuch as these species and subspecies can only be distinguished microscopically, this handbook treats the disease as one irrespective of which subspecies is the cause.

The disease, originally native to the Douglas-fir regions of western North America, is now also found in eastern North America and Europe. In California, Oregon, and Washington it appears sporadically in most native Douglas-fir stands. *R. pseudotsugae* is found only on 1-year-old needles, while *R. weirii* is found on older needles as well. A single attack usually results in only partial defoliation of the host. Trees subjected to several consecutive years of attack may be completely defoliated and killed or severely restricted in growth. Such damage is rare in natural stands, but is not uncommon on sites where the host is not well adapted. The greatest financial damage occurs when Christmas tree plantations are attacked, because defoliation makes them unsalable for a few years. This disease is most severe on younger trees up to pole size. Mature trees when attacked usually are only affected slightly.

Disease cycle—Fruiting bodies appear on the undersurface of needles infected the previous year and mature and release ascospores in May or June. These spores, carried by air currents, land on and infect the current-year's developing needles. Moist conditions favor infection. The fungus continues to develop in the newly infected needles that summer and fall. The first symptoms appear early that first winter as slightly yellowish spots at the site of infection. During the winter these spots become larger and more distinct. By spring the spots have changed to a deep red-brown color, and many of the spots have merged. In late spring, elliptical fruiting bodies (apothecia) appear on the undersurface of the needle on either side of the midrib. These mature and sporulate in May or June, and the infected needles are cast during the following summer. It is suggested that those subspecies appearing on needles 2 years old or older attack the current-year's needles but have a 2- to 3-year developmental cycle.

Field identification—The best time for identifying this disease is in late spring, when the needles are still retained and the red-brown needle spots and developing fruiting bodies are visible. During the summer, generally all of the needles are cast, and the only field

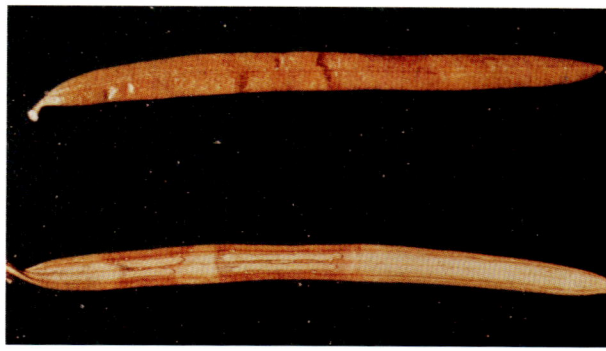

Figure 2-5—
Douglas-fir needle cast caused by Rhabdocline *spp. The light colored fruiting bodies of* R. pseudotsugae *are located in the red-brown spots on the underside of an infected needle, as shown on the lower needle.*

symptom is the absence of needles of a single year's growth of the host.

The disease is characterized by the red-brown needle spots and the long brown cushion-like fruiting bodies (apothecia) which develop on either side of the mid-rib on the underside of the infected needles (fig. 2-5). At maturity, the epidermis covering the fruiting bodies splits irregularly, exposing an orange to orange-brown spore-bearing surface.

TRUE FIR NEEDLE DISEASES

A^1 On bristlecone fir .... B
A^2 On other firs C
B^1 Fruiting bodies brownish-black, large, extending down the middle of the needle for almost its whole length .... *Lirula nervisequia*
B^2 Fruiting bodies grayish-black, elliptical, appearing in two rows, on each side of mid-rib .... *Lophodermium decorum*
C^1 Fruiting bodies on needles of all ages, appearing as oval disc-like structures breaking through the lower epidermis in two rows, one on either side of the mid-rib snow mold .... *Phacidium abietis*
C^2 Fruiting bodies brownish-black, large, elongate extending down center of lower surface of 2-year-old or older needles .... D
D^1 Pycnidial fruiting structures appear as a single brownish line down the center groove of upper surface of needle .... *Lirula abietis-concoloris*
D^2 Pycnidia on needles tan to light brown appearing as two wrinkles or rows, one on each wing, along the upper needle surface .... *Virgella robusta*

Figure 2-6—*Fir needle cast caused by* Lirula abietis-concoloris *killed the needles on this young white fir.*

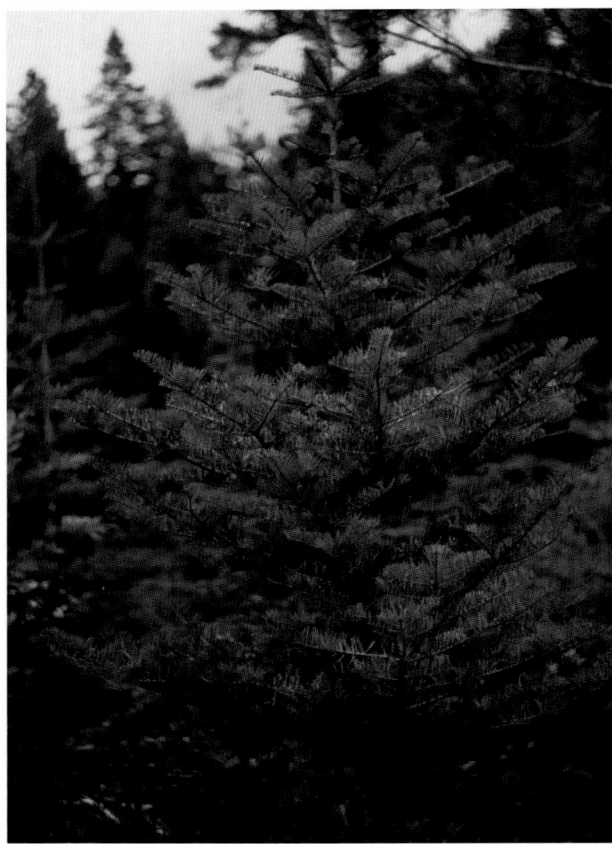

True Fir Needle Casts
Lirula abietis-concoloris
Virgella robusta

Hosts—In the western United States, *Lirula abietis-concoloris* and *Virgella robusta* have been found on white, grand, noble, Pacific silver, and California red firs.

Distribution and damage—Both fungi are found throughout western North America, generally wherever their hosts occur. As with many other needle casts, they appear sporadically and in many areas infrequently.

As a rule, these diseases are of little economic importance in the forest. Since they occur sporadically and attack only 1-year's complement of needles, they seldom kill a significant proportion of the host's foliage. Only if several successive years of infection were to occur would they defoliate trees and greatly affect host growth and vigor. Their most serious effect is damage to Christmas trees. The unsightly browning of the infected needles makes the tree unsalable (fig. 2-6).

Disease cycle—Little information is available on the life history of these fungi. Field studies indicate a 2-year life cycle, with infection occurring on young, developing needles during periods of rainfall. Fruiting structures mature on these needles in spring the second year after infection.

Field identification—Both fungi may be identified by the presence of their elongate, dark brown or black fruiting bodies (hysterothecia) (figs. 2-7, 2-8) on 2-year-old or older straw-colored needles. These fruiting bodies extend down the center of the lower needle surface for almost its full length. Infection is usually confined to 1 year's complement of needles.

These fungi may be distinguished from each other by the arrangement of pycnidial fruiting bodies on the upper surface of the needles. In *V. robusta,* the pycnidia form two distinct light brown rows or wrinkles—one on each wing of the infected needle (fig. 2-7). In *L. abietis-concoloris*, the pycnidia form a single brown line or occasionally a double row of dots in the groove down the center of the needle (fig. 2-8).

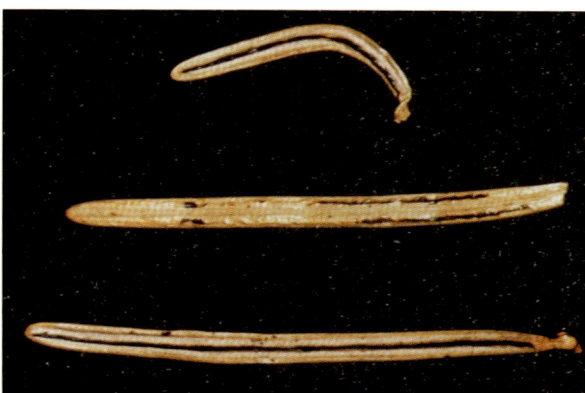

Figure 2-7—*The needles of white fir are infected by a needle cast fungus,* Virgella robusta. *The needles on the top and bottom show the heavy dark hysterothecium on the lower surface of the needle, and the needle in the center shows the two rows of concolorous to brown pycnidia on the upper needle surface.*

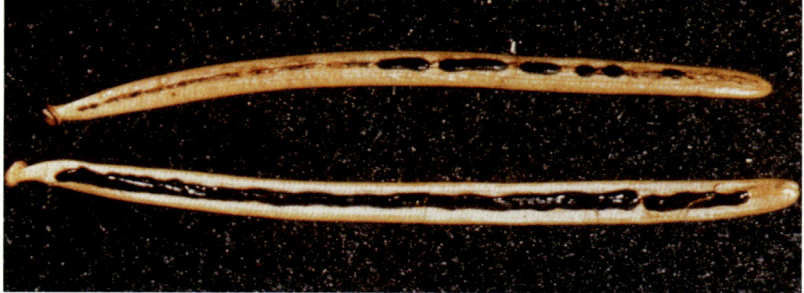

Figure 2-8—*Conspicuous fruiting bodies of* Lirula abietis-concoloris *develop on infected needles of white fir. The needle on the bottom shows the heavy dark hysterothecium on the lower needle surface. On the upper needle, the pycnidia appear as a thin, brown line on the upper needle surface.*

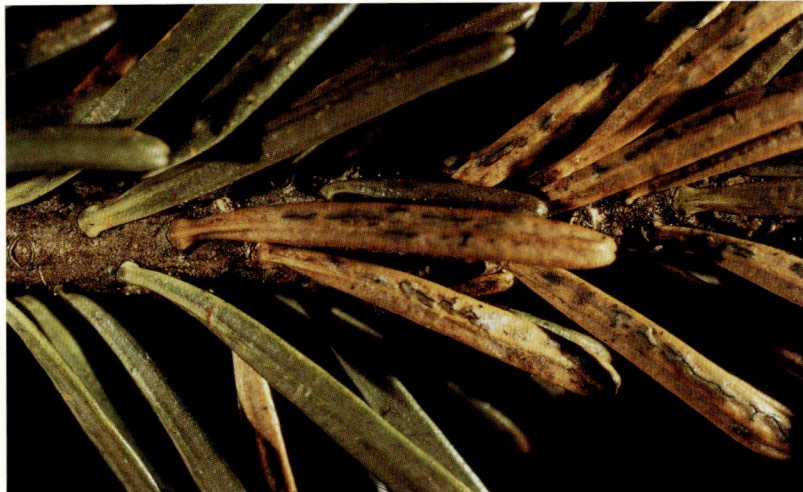

Figure 2-9—*The dark fruiting bodies of* Lophodermium decorum *are readily seen on the lower surface of an infected needle of alpine fir.*

Bristlecone Fir Needle Cast
Lirula nervisequia ssp. *conspicua*

A disease similar to the other true fir needle casts and caused by *Lirula nervisequia* is found on bristlecone fir in Monterey County, CA. The fruiting bodies are brownish-black, large, elongate structures extending down the middle of the undersurface of the needle for most of its length. This fungus appears rarely and does little damage.

Lophodermium decorum

In the western United States, *Lophodermium decorum* is found on shaded and weakened needles of grand fir. This rare fungus is easily differentiated from the other true fir needle casts by its two rows of short, elliptical, brown to grayish-black, fruiting bodies on the lower needle surface, one row on each side of the mid-rib (fig. 2-9). A similar but as yet unnamed species of *Lophodermium* has been reported on bristlecone fir.

Snow Blight
Phacidium abietis

Snow blight caused by the fungus *Phacidium abietis* has been found on the needles of white fir in the southern Cascade Mountains and the northern Sierra Nevada in California. At times, it has reached epidemic proportions in northern Idaho and eastern Oregon, killing reproduction of grand fir, subalpine fir, and Douglas-fir. The fungus attacks needles of all ages during winter while they are under the snow. After the snow has melted, the infected needles remain on the

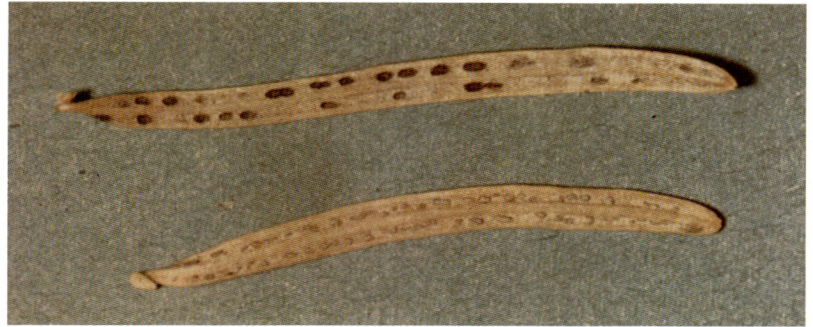

Figure 2-10—*Snow blight of white fir caused by* Phacidium abietis. *The dark brown oval fruiting bodies are arranged in two rows along the lower needle surface.*

tree and turn brown. Only those needles covered by snow during winter are attacked. In summer and fall, dark brown, round to oval, disc-like fruiting bodies break through the lower epidermis of the needle. The fruiting bodies are arranged in two rows, one on either side of the mid-rib (fig. 2-10). They mature and release spores from August to October. The following year the needles remain attached to the host and turn gray. The fruiting bodies fall away, leaving a cavity in the lower needle surface much like the one that occurs in the cedar leaf blight.

PINE NEEDLE DISEASES

A^1 Infection perennial in twigs, resulting in necrotic flecks in inner bark; in a red flagging of almost all 1-year-old needles on infected twigs in the spring; and a brooming and upturning of infected twigs .... *Elytroderma deformans*

A^2 Infection not perennial in twigs; separate infection of each needle required; no brooming .... B

B^1 Infected needles with bright red bands or spots with black fruiting bodies on 1-, 2-, or 3-year-old needles .... *Mycospharella pini*

B^2 Infected needles not as above C

C^1 Fruiting bodies on infected needles exposed by the splitting of the epidermis along stomatal lines and tearing at the ends of the fruiting body to form two door-like epidermal flaps that remain hinged at the side; exposed brown spore layer .... *Cyclaneusma niveum*

C^2 Fruiting bodies opening by a narrow slit, elliptical to elongate, black to brown .... D

D^1 Host in the white pine group .... E

D^2 Host in the hard pine group I

E¹	Fruiting body light brown to concolorous with the needle surface .... *Lophodermella arcuata*
E²	Fruiting body black .... F
F¹	Fruiting body shiny black with irregular black crust-like growth of fungus tissue .... *Bifusella linearis*
F²	Fruiting body without associated crust-like growth .... G
G¹	Fruiting bodies shiny black, elliptical, associated pycnidia brown, on needles of singleleaf pinyon pine .... *Bifusella pini*
G²	Fruiting bodies large and black, associated pycnidia black, on whitebark and limber pines .... *Bifusella saccata*
G³	On other white pines .... H
H¹	Fruiting bodies shiny black, elliptical occurring subcuticularly in groups on outer surface of needles; group of fruiting bodies separated from adjacent groups by distinct black lines bisecting the needle .... *Lophodermium nitens*
H²	Fruiting bodies dull to shiny black, elliptical, occurring in rows on all surfaces of 3-year or older needles. Infected needles often remain on tree and turn gray .... *Lophodermium pinastri* complex
I¹	Fruiting body light brown to concolorous with needle surface .... J
I²	Fruiting body black .... K
J¹	Fruiting bodies oval and concolorous, on ponderosa and lodgepole pine .... *Lophodermella cerina*
J²	Fruiting bodies elongate, concolorous to brown on ponderosa and knobcone pine .... *Lophodermella morbida*
K¹	Fruiting bodies often found in dead areas of live green needles L
K²	Fruiting bodies found on completely dead or faded needles .... M
L¹	Fruiting bodies in dead areas of live green needles of *Pinus radiata* or *P. attenuata* .... either *Davisomycella lacrimiformis* or *Davisomycella limitata*
L²	On lodgepole pine, fruiting bodies in dead areas and separated from green areas by an orange-brown band that remains even after the whole needle dies .... *Davisomycella montana*
M¹	Fruiting bodies, elongate, black .... N
M²	Fruiting bodies elliptical, dull to shiny black, occurring in rows on all surfaces of 3-year-old needles. Infected needles often remain on the tree and turn gray .... *Lophodermium pinastri*

N¹ Fruiting bodies elongate, black, wide, one-third to one-half the width of the needle, variable in length, occurring on lighter-colored zones on dead 3-year-old needles .... *Davisomycella medusa*
N² Fruiting bodies elongate, thin, occurring on dead 1-year-old needles, not found in lighter-colored zone .... *Elytroderma deformans*

Elytroderma Disease
Elytroderma deformans

Hosts—Elytroderma disease of pines caused by the fungus *Elytroderma deformans* is considered to be the most important needle cast of ponderosa and Jeffrey pines in western North America. Its perennial nature and capacity to infect the host twigs, which is unique among the needle casts, enable it to maintain its populations even under adverse environmental conditions.

Although mainly a disease of ponderosa and Jeffrey pines, elytroderma disease has been found on Coulter, knobcone, lodgepole, and pinyon pines.

Distribution and damage—Elytroderma disease is limited to North America mainly west of the Rockies. It is scattered throughout most of the pine forests of California, Oregon, and Washington. For the most part, the disease occurs only in forests above 3,500 feet (1,067 m) elevation in Washington and above 5,000 to 6,000 feet (1,524 to 1,829 m) in Oregon and California. The disease has reached epidemic proportions in certain specific environments, such as around lakes and along stream bottoms. Its concentration around lakes such as Lake Tahoe in California has considerable effect on the appearance of high-value recreational sites because of the defoliation and tree death it causes.

This fungus causes the premature death of 1-year-old needles and a brooming and deformation of infected twigs and branches. The effect of the disease depends on the proportion of the host's crown that is diseased. There is little effect upon the host until more than two-fifths of the twigs are blighted. The disease's impact is greatest on seedlings, saplings, and poles with poor crowns. Although this disease directly kills mature trees infrequently, moderate to severe infection reduces growth and vigor and thus predisposes the host to other diseases and to bark beetle attack.

Disease cycle—Spores of the causal fungus are released in late spring and early summer from fruiting bodies borne on infected needles. Air currents carry the spores to the young current-year's needles of a susceptible host. Under conditions of rain or free moisture, the spores germinate and infect the young needles. The fungus spreads throughout the needles and into the twigs without initially killing the needles. The following spring the infected needles die and turn red brown, and fruiting bodies that mature in spring and summer begin to form. The infection within the twigs spreads into the growing tips and buds, where it causes a brooming and deformation of future growth. New needles formed each year from infected buds are infected as they form. These needles stay green their first year, die in spring of their second year, and produce fruiting bodies. Thus, *E. deformans* produces a new crop of spores each year for many years from the same infection.

Field identification—Elytroderma disease is relatively easy to identify in the field. The most conspicuous symptoms are reddening of the infected foliage in spring, witches-brooms, necrotic flecks in the inner bark of older infected twigs, and elongate, black fruiting bodies on dead needles (fig. 2-11a,b,c). The infected needles lose their bright red-brown color gradually through the summer. The brooms tend to be more compact and globose than those caused by dwarf mistletoe, and the ends of the twigs turn up. The brown necrotic flecks in the inner bark of twigs infected for more than 3 years are quite characteristic. Their presence is one of the best evidences for confirming this disease. The fruiting structures of the fungus that appear on infected needles in late spring are elongate, narrow, dull black, and scattered on all surfaces of the needle (fig. 2-11d).

Red Band Needle Blight
Mycospharella (Scirrhia) pini
(Dothistroma septospora)

Hosts—*Mycospharella pini* (imperfect stage—*Dothistroma septospora*) attacks some 30 species, varieties, or hybrids of pines. In western North America, it has been found on Bishop, ponderosa, western white, lodgepole, knobcone, and Monterey pines and the Monterey X knobcone hybrid.

Distribution and damage—Red band needle blight is distributed worldwide. In western North America, it has been reported from north coastal California north into British Columbia and east to Idaho. This disease is considered to be the most destructive needle disease of pines throughout the world. Its discovery along the Pacific Coast in the 1960's, therefore, aroused considerable concern. But for the most part, it was found to be damaging in only a few localized infection centers along the coast. The fungus attacks the needles of susceptible pines, causing them to die and drop off. Needles of all ages are susceptible. Under favorable environmental conditions, this disease can completely defoliate the host in a few weeks and eventually kill the infected trees. Monterey pine, although severely affected when young, becomes resistant to this disease after it becomes 20 to 30 years old.

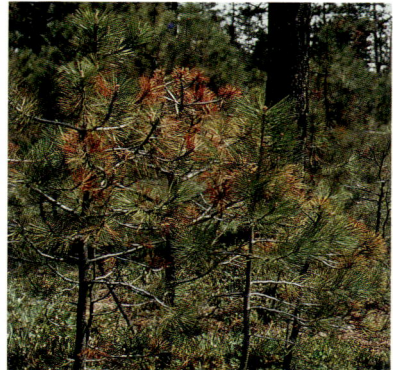
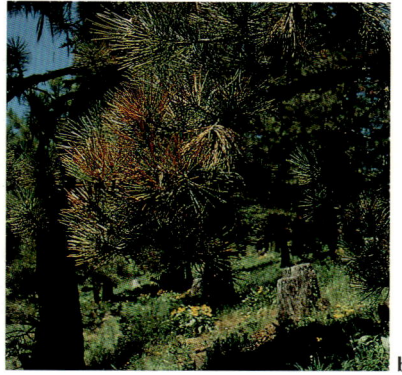
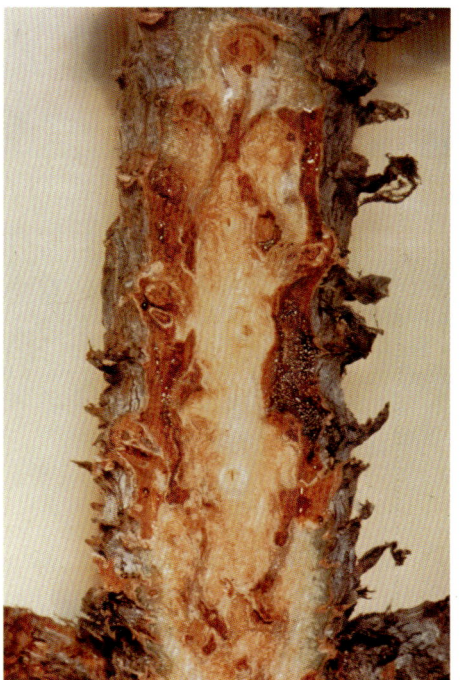

Figure 2-11—Seedlings infected by elytroderma disease show the stunting and reddening of last year's infected needles (**a**). Conspicuous brooms often develop on branches infected by Elytroderma deformans (**b**). Brown necrotic flecks appear in the inner bark of an older twig of ponderosa pine infected with elytroderma disease (**c**). The fruiting bodies of E. deformans appearing in June on dying, brown needles are elongate, narrow, dull black, and scattered on all needle surfaces (**d**).

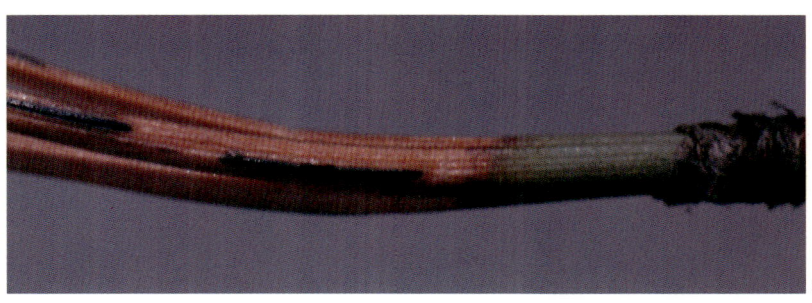

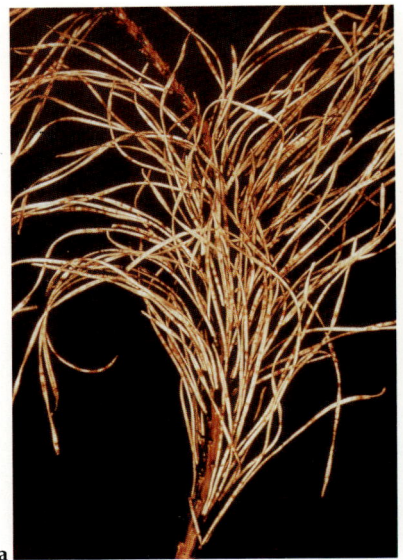 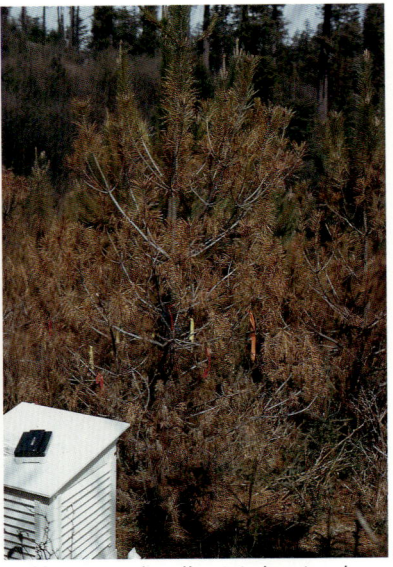

Figure 2-12—*The red band needle blight caused by* Mycospharella pini *showing the red banding around the infected needles* (**a**). *A young Monterey pine showing severe needle disease caused by* Mycospharella pini (**b**).

Disease cycle—Fruiting bodies (pycnidia) are produced in abundance on infected needles. In the presence of free water, these pycnidia liberate spores that are splashed or blown to uninfected needles. Under moist conditions, the spores infect the new needles. The fungus grows within the needle tissue, killing the distal portion of the needle. Again, under favorable conditions, new pycnidia and spores are produced. Dead needles remain attached to the host and produce spores for about a year.

Field identification—The first noticeable symptoms are yellow to tan spots appearing at the site of infection. These spots turn a brownish red and enlarge to produce the characteristic red band around the needle (fig. 2-12a). This red band on the infected needles is diagnostic for this disease. Small black fruiting bodies develop in the center of the red bands. The portion of the needle distal to the infection dies, although the uninfected base of the needle may remain green for some time. Often nearly all the foliage on a tree becomes infected (fig. 2-12b). Trees infected for several years often exhibit a "lion's tail" appearance, with only a few needles remaining at the ends of branches.

Sugar Pine Needle Cast
Lophodermella arcuata

Hosts—The sugar pine needle cast caused by the fungus *Lophodermella arcuata* has been reported on western white pine

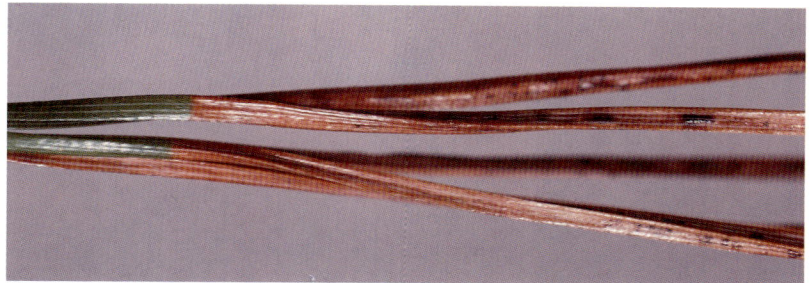

Figure 2-13—*Dying needles of sugar pine showing the black fruiting bodies of* Lophodermella arcuata *on the brown portion of the needles.*

from Idaho and Oregon and on sugar pine in California and Oregon.

Distribution and damage—This disease is found generally throughout western North America where sugar and western white pines grow. It appears more prevalent in Oregon and northern California than in southern California, where it is found only in canyon bottoms. This disease attacks only the current-year's needles, and a single attack results in only partial defoliation of the host. Repeated consecutive infections, as have occurred in certain local areas, have led to reduced tree growth and vigor and occasional tree mortality.

Disease cycle—This fungus infects newly developing foliage. Infected foliage remains green an entire year until the following spring (April to May), when the needles die back from the tips and turn brown. This browning occurs before bud break, giving heavily infected trees a scorched appearance. At this time, there is no sign of the fruiting bodies. Concolorous fruiting bodies appear in mid-June and mature in July and August on the dead portions of the needles (fig. 2-13). The needles are cast in mid to late summer after spores are discharged.

Field identification—This disease can be identified in the field by the dark brown to concolorous, elongate to elliptical, fruiting structures, which develop on all surfaces of the previous year's dead and dying needles.

Bifusella linearis

The fungus *Bifusella linearis* causes a needle cast of 2- to 3-year-old needles of western white, limber, and whitebark pines in the western United States. This disease ranges south from British Columbia to the higher mountains of California and east into Idaho. Because of its limited distribution, small host range, and restriction to older needles, the fungus is not considered to be a serious pest. The fungus forms shiny black, elongate, fruiting bodies of variable lengths on the surface of 2- to 3-year-old needles. Frequently associated with the fruiting bodies are black crust-like growths of fungus tissue (sometimes including pycnidia) that are irregular in size and outline (fig. 2-14). These crust-like formations are the most distinctive characteristic of this disease in the field.

Singleleaf Pine Needle Cast
Bifusella pini

Bifusella pini occurs only on singleleaf pinyon pine in western Nevada and southern California. It forms long, shiny, black, elliptical, fruiting bodies (hysterothecia) on all surfaces of needles 4 years and older (fig. 2-15) as well as pycnidia, which vary from brown dots to long, irregular, brown blotches on needles 3 years of age or older. This disease is seldom damaging.

Bifusella saccata

The fungus *Bifusella saccata* has been found on whitebark pine in California and limber and pinyon pines in Colorado. It has been reported only from elevations above 9,000 feet (2,743 m) in the southern Sierra Nevada. Because of its limited distribution and small host range, this disease is not considered to be economically important. This fungus forms large, long, shiny, black fruiting bodies on the dead tips of green needles (fig. 2-16).

Lophodermium nitens

Lophodermium nitens is found in both eastern and western North America. In California, it is common on the needles of sugar pine, fairly common on western white pine, and rare on whitebark pine. The fruiting bodies are shiny black, elliptical, blister-like structures on the outer surface of the needles. They mature on dead fallen needles and occasionally on the tips of partially green, attached needles. These fruiting bodies occur singly or in clusters. Each cluster is separated from adjacent clusters above and below by a very distinct black line bisecting the needle and along which the needle readily breaks (fig. 2-17).

Lophodermium pinastri complex

In the western United States, several similar but different species of needle cast fungi have in the past been lumped together and all called *Lophodermium pinastri*. This treatment of several species as one has caused much confusion in understanding the taxonomy, biology, and distribution of *L. pinastri* and its close associates. The taxonomy of this complex was recently revised and is now thought to contain the following four species: *L. pinastri, L. pini-excelsae, L. conigenum,* and *L. seditiosum.*

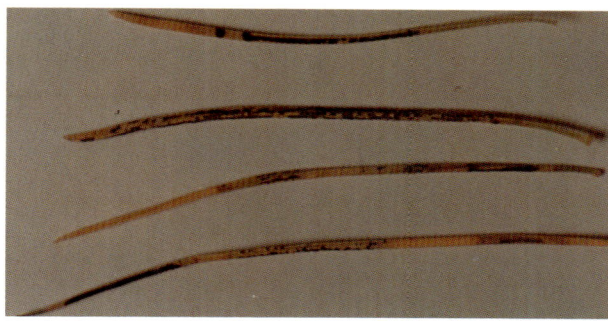

Figure 2-14—*The fruiting bodies of* Bifusella linearis *on the needles of limber pine. Note the black crustlike formation with its irregular margin.*

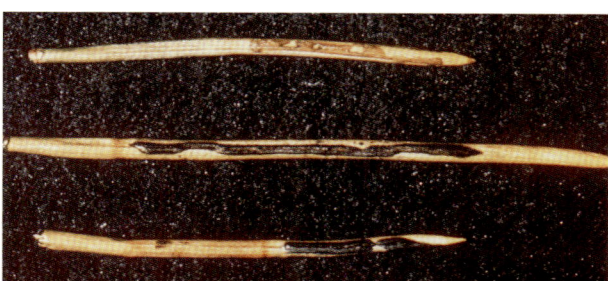

Figure 2-15—*The long shiny black fruiting bodies of singleleaf pinyon needle cast caused by* Bifusella pini *appear on the two needles of singleleaf pinyon pine on the Bottom and the brown pycnidia on the needle on the top.*

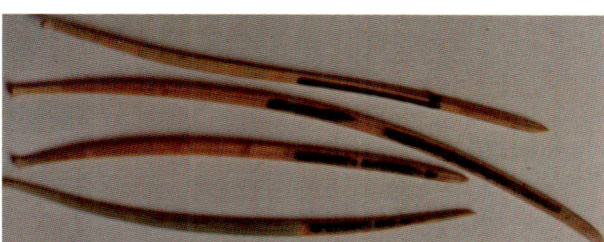

Figure 2-16—*The fruiting bodies of* Bifusella saccata *on whitebark pine.*

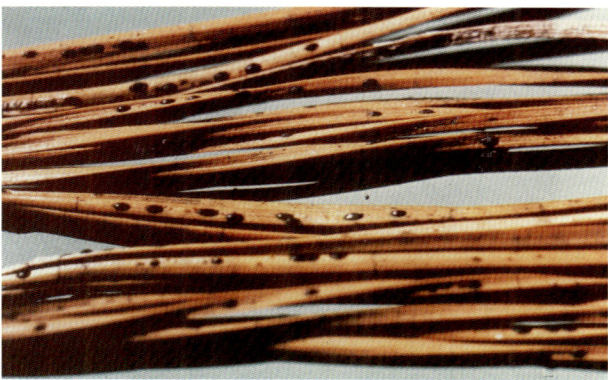

Figure 2-17—Lophodermium nitens *on the needles of sugar pine. Note the shiny black blister-like elliptical fruiting bodies and the fine black lines that cross the needles.*

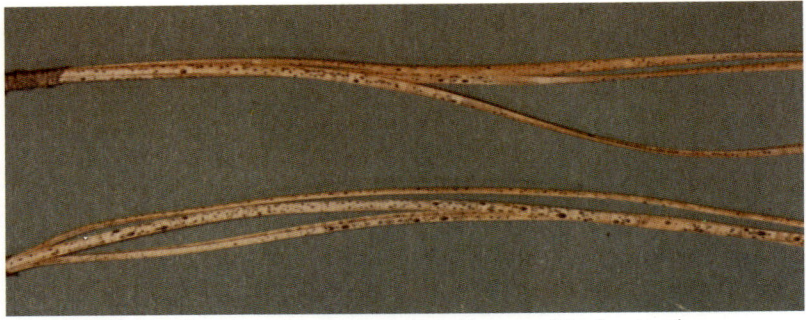

Figure 2-18—*Needles of ponderosa pine infected by one of the fungi in the* Lophodermium pinastri *complex. The fruiting bodies are small, black, irregular in size, and scattered over the needle surface.*

The needle diseases caused by these species of *Lophodermium* are found in the United States and throughout the world. They are found on many species of pine. In the western United States, they have been found on Digger, Jeffrey, Coulter, knobcone, lodgepole, Monterey, ponderosa, sugar, western white, and whitebark pines. Because the available host range for *L. pinastri* was developed before the recent taxonomic revision and this revision was based solely on Scotch pine as the host, we can say little about the host ranges for each of the species in the *L. pinastri* complex. Three of the species, *L. pinastri*, *L. pini-excelsae,* and *L. seditiosum,* are listed as occurring on Scotch pine on the west coast of North America. The fourth species, *L. conigenum,* is listed as occurring in Michigan. New host and geographic ranges for these four fungi will have to be determined using the new descriptions in the recent taxonomic revision. The main characters used to distinguish and separate these four species are (1) position of the fruiting body in relation to the needle epidermis, (2) the presence, number, and color of stromatic lines through the needles, and (3) the color of the lips at the ascocarp opening (table 1).

The diseases that are caused by this complex appear to be common and usually do little or no damage to their hosts except in some cases in which trees have been planted off-site. In general, the fruiting bodies of most of these fungi appear on all surfaces of 3-year-old or older needles as dull to shining black, elliptical structures that tend to occur in lines or rows (fig. 2-18). Mature fruiting bodies open by a conspicuous longitudinal slit. The infected needles often remain on the tree for several years after dying.

Lophodermella cerina

The fungus *Lophodermella cerina* causes a needle blight of lodgepole and ponderosa pines in California from Modoc County south to Fresno County. The disease has been severe and damaging in

Table 1—Useful taxonomic characters for identification of the four species in the *Lophodermium pinastri* complex

Species	Color	Fruiting body Position	Lip color	Stromatic lines
L. pinastri	More than 50% black	Subcuticular	Usually red lines	Many black
L. pini-excelsae	More than 50% black	Subcuticular	Gray lines	Few black
L. conigenum	Less than 25% black	Mostly subepidermal	Gray	Brown
L. seditiosum	All grey	Completely subepidermal	Hyaline, green or blue	Brown

certain areas for several years. The fruiting bodies of this fungus are short, oval, light-brown to buff structures, and they are easily overlooked on necrotic pine needles. At first, they are slightly darker and then the same color as the needle spot on which they occur. They develop in groups in buff to tawny waxy spots on live green or dead, reddish brown needles. The short concolorous fruiting body is the most distinctive characteristic of this fungus.

Lophodermella morbida

Hosts—*Lophodermella morbida* is found on ponderosa pine in Oregon and Washington and knobcone pine in northern California.

Distribution and damage—This disease is found only in the mild, moist climate west of the crest of the Cascade Mountains in Oregon and Washington and the western slopes of the Coast Range of Northern California. It attacks the current-year's needles, which become necrotic in late summer or early fall and then drop off the second summer. A single year's attack results in only partial defoliation, but repeated attacks, as have occurred in ponderosa pine in Oregon, result in complete defoliation and death of the tree (fig. 2-19). This pathogen has been described as highly aggressive.

Disease cycle—Needles of the current year are infected in June and become necrotic as early as the end of July. Pycnidia begin to appear in October, and light brown hysterothecia are faintly evident by mid-November. Ascospores are mature and ready for discharge by mid-June of the following year. Moist conditions are necessary for ascospore release and infection. Infected needles are cast shortly thereafter.

Field identification—This disease is characterized by light brown (concolorous), immature hysterothecia that darken as they mature.

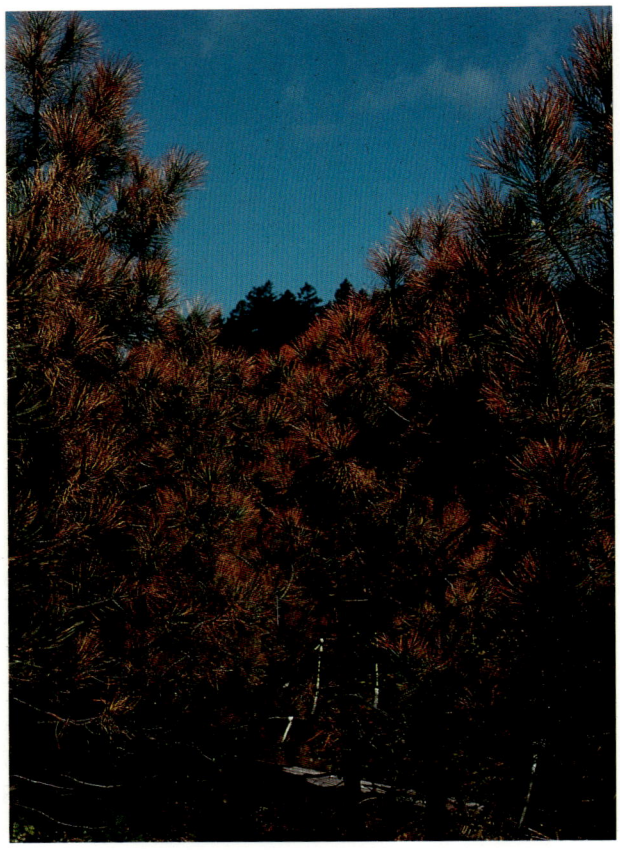

Figure 2-19— *Ponderosa pines on some sites in western Oregon and Washington can be severely defoliated by* Lophodermella morbida.

These elongate fruiting bodies (1 to 6 mm long) occur in an interrupted linear or occasionally double-rowed series that may extend the full length of the needle (fig. 2-20). The pycnidia are light brown, round to elongate structures, 0.25 mm in diameter and up to 1.5 mm long.

Davisomycella limitata
Davisomycella lacrimiformis

The fungi *Davisomycella limitata* and *D. lacrimiformis* cause identical diseases of Monterey pine. The latter also attacks knobcone pine. The fruiting bodies are black, elliptical to oblong, often confluent and scattered on dead areas on still green living needles. *D. limitata* has been found in central coastal California. *D. lacrimiformis* has been reported from the coastal mountains of California and Oregon. Both diseases appear to be of little economic importance.

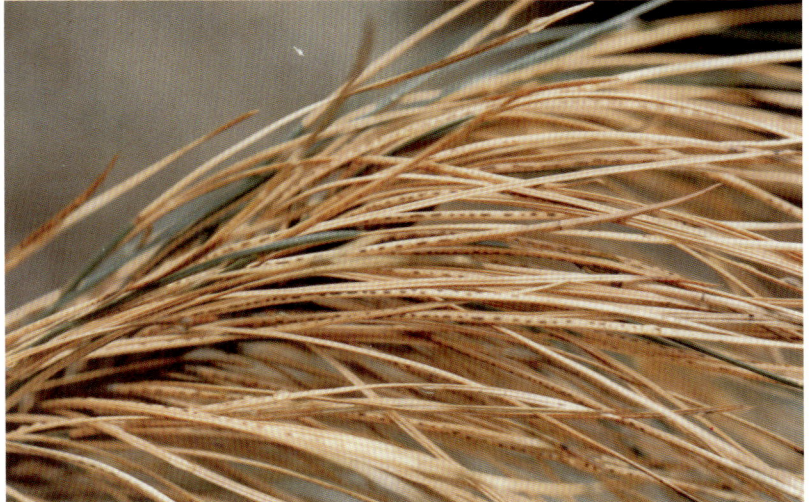

Figure 2-20—Lophodermella morbida *on ponderosa pine. The light to dark brown fruiting bodies occur in rows along the infected needles.*

Lodgepole Pine Needle Cast
Davisomycella montana

The lodgepole pine needle cast caused by the fungus *Davisomycella montana* has been reported in Idaho, Oregon, and California. Although widespread throughout California, the disease does not appear to cause much damage to its host except in a few localized areas. This disease is characterized by the appearance of fruiting bodies on dead brown areas on 2-year-old needles. The dead areas are frequently found on green needles and are separated from the green tissues by an orange-brown zone, or band. This orange band remains visible even after the needle dies and turns brown. The fruiting bodies appear as shiny, black, raised, elliptical blisters scattered on all surfaces of the dead areas (fig. 2-21). These fruiting bodies mature during the period from July to September.

Medusa Needle Blight
Davisomycella medusa

Hosts—The medusa needle blight is found on lodgepole, Jeffrey, and ponderosa pines.

Distribution and damage—This needle disease is widely distributed throughout the ponderosa and Jeffrey pine forests east of the Cascades in Washington, Oregon, and northern California. It becomes a serious pest in local areas on individual trees, often causing a marked decrease in growth. It characteristically occurs in relatively

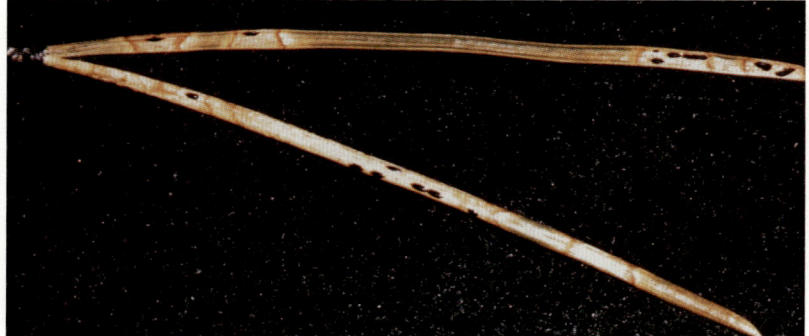

Figure 2-21—*The shiny black fruiting bodies of lodgepole pine needle cast caused by Davisomycella montana are grouped in the light straw-colored areas on needles bordered by an orange-brown band.*

pure open stands and tends to be most pronounced on medium-to-poor sites. It also tends to become more intense after a drought.

Life cycle—Fruiting bodies (hysterothecia) mature on infected needles in June, and spore discharge occurs in summer and fall. These spores are carried by the wind to nearby pines, where they infect the current-year's needles. The disease remains latent for 2 to 4 years within the infected needles before a greenish-white fading of the infected foliage occurs. The fruiting bodies of the fungus then appear on the affected needles as elongate, blackish raised blisters.

Field identification—The best time for identifying this disease is in late spring to early summer. The elongate, black, raised, fruiting bodies are one-third to one-half the width of the needle and variable in length (fig. 2-22). They appear on greenish-white to straw-colored zones that are lighter in color than the rest of the needle. These zones, occupying one-fifth to one-third the length of the needle, may occur on any portion of the needle, but are found more commonly near the base.

Cyclaneusma niveum

Cyclaneusma niveum causes a minor needle disease of some pines in the western United States, particularly Monterey, lodgepole, ponderosa, and Jeffrey pines. In the eastern United States and Europe, it is a more virulent pathogen and causes extensive defoliation of pines, especially Scotch pines grown for Christmas trees. The fungus spreads by spores and infects young foliage during periods of rain. Light-colored fruiting bodies develop on all surfaces of a needle about a year after infection. Damage is of little consequence in the forest environment, but pines grown for Christmas trees or ornamentals could lose some foliage. Trees are not killed by this disease.

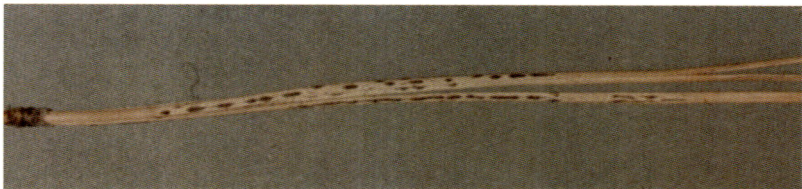

Figure 2-22—*Medusa needle blight caused by* Davisomycella medusa *infects needles of ponderosa pine. Elongate, raised, black fruiting bodies appear in the light-colored zones of the infected needles and are more numerous towards the base of the needle.*

SELECTED REFERENCES

Boyce, J.S. 1940. A needle-cast of Douglas-fir associated with *Adelopus gaumanni*. Phytopathology 30:649–659.
Boyce, J.S. 1961. Forest Pathology, 3d ed. New York: McGraw-Hill Book Co. : 153–193.
Brandt, R.W. 1960. The R*habdocline* needle cast of Douglas-fir. Tech. Publ. 84. Syracuse, NY: New York State University College of Forestry. 66 p.
Childs, T.W. 1968. Elytroderma disease of ponderosa pine in the Pacific Northwest. Res. Pap. PNW-69. Portland, OR: U.S. Department of Agriculture, Forest Service, Pacific Northwest Forest and Range Experiment Station. 45 p.
Darker, G.D. 1932. The Hypodermataceae of conifers. Jamaica Plain, MA: Arnold Arboretum Harvard Press. 131 p.
Darker, G.D. 1966. A revision of the genera of the Hypodermataceae. Canadian Journal of Botany 45:1399–1444.
Funk, A. 1985. Foliar fungi of western trees. Victoria, BC. Canadian Forestry Research Service, Pacific Forest Research Centre. 159 p.
Funk, A.; Parker, A.K. 1966. *Scirrhia pini* N. Sp., the perfect state of *Dothistroma pini* Hulbary. Canadian Journal of Botany 44:1171–1176.
Minter, D.W.; Staley J.M.; Millar C.S. 1978. Four species of *Lophodermium* on *Pinus sylvestris*. Transactions of the British Mycological Society 71:295–301.
Morton, H.L.; Patton, R.F. 1970. Swiss needle cast of Douglas-fir in the Lake States. Plant Disease Reporter 54:612–616.
Parker, A.K. 1967. Rhabdocline needle cast of Douglas-fir, *Rhabdocline pseudotsugae*. In: Important forest insect and diseases of mutual concern to Canada, the United States, and Mexico. Ottawa: Queen's Printer and Controller of Stationery. 207 p.
Parker, A.K.; Colis, D.G. 1966. Dothistroma needle blight of pines in British Columbia. Forestry Chronicle 2:160–161.
Parker, A.K.; Reid J. 1969. The genus *Rhabdocline* Syd. Canadian Journal of Botany 47:1533–1545.
Peace, T.R. 1962. Pathology of trees and shrubs. London: Oxford University, Clarendon Press. 753 p.
Reid, J.; Cain, R.F. 1962. Studies on the organisms associated with "snow blight" of conifers in North America. II. Some species of the genera *Phadicum, Lophophacidium, Sarcotrichila,* and *Hemiphacidium*. Mycologia 54:481–497.
Scharpf, R.F. 1990. Life cycle and epidemiology of *Elytroderma deformans* on pines in California. In: Merrill, W.; Ostry, M.E., eds. Recent research on foliage diseases, conference proceedings; 1989 May 29-June 2; Carlisle, PA. Gen. Tech. Rep. WO-56. Washington, DC: U.S. Department of Agriculture, Forest Service: 7–12.
Scharpf, R.F.; Bega, R.V. 1981. Elytroderma disease reduces growth and vigor, increases mortality of Jeffrey pines at Lake Tahoe Basin, California. Res. Paper PSW-155. Berkeley, CA: U.S. Department of Agriculture, Forest Service, Pacific Southwest Forest and Range Experiment Station. 6 p.
Scharpf, R.F.; Staley, J.; Hawksworth, F.G. 1970. A needle cast, the first known disease of bristlecone fir in California. Plant Disease Reporter 54:275–277.

Simms, H.R. 1967. On the ecology of *Herpotrichia nigra*. Mycologia 49:902–909.
Staley, J.M.; Bynum, H.H. 1972. A new *Lophodermella* on *Pinus ponderosa* and *P. attenuata*. Mycologia 64:722–726.
Sturgis, W.C. 1913. *Herpotrichia* and *Neopeckia* on conifers. Phytopathology 3:152–158.
Thyr, B.D.; Shaw, C.G. 1964. Identity of the fungus causing red band disease on pines. Mycologia 56:103–109.
Wagener, W.W. 1959. The effect of a western needle fungus (*Hypoderma medusa* Dearn.) on pines and its significance in forest management. Journal of Forestry 57:561–564.
Wagener, W.W. 1967. Red band needle blight of pines: a tentative appraisal for California. Res. Note PSW-153. Berkeley, CA: Department of Agriculture, Forest Service, Pacific Southwest Forest and Range Experiment Station. 6 p.

CHAPTER 3   Cankers, Diebacks, and Galls

Robert F. Scharpf
Research Scientist Emeritus, formerly Project Leader, Disease Research, and Principal Plant Pathologist, Pacific Southwest Research Station, Forest Service, U.S. Department of Agriculture, Albany, CA.

INTRODUCTION

This chapter describes the tree diseases known as cankers, diebacks, and galls. The term *canker* as discussed here refers to any localized necrotic area or spot on branches or trunks of trees. Most cankers are caused by certain species of fungi, but some by adverse climate (see chapter 1). *Dieback* refers to rapid girdling or tip killing of twigs and branches that is caused mainly by canker fungi. *Galls*, commonly called burls, are pronounced swellings on branches, trunks, and leaves caused by fungi, bacteria, mistletoes, insects, or other agents.

In many instances, initial infection by a fungus results in a localized canker that subsequently girdles a branch, causing dieback. Often dead branches are the only symptoms of the disease—particularly in small branches that are girdled and killed quickly with no apparent canker development. In other instances, both dieback and cankers occur on the same tree.

Cankers vary considerably in appearance and occurrence. They may be sunken or slightly swollen, circular or elongate in shape. Some show little or no healing, whereas others are progressively callused-over so that concentric rings are formed. Cankers are either *annual* or *perennial*.

Annual cankers occur sporadically—for 1 year or one season only. They result from unusually severe weather conditions (chapter 1) or a particular sequence of climatic conditions that favor the attack of trees by certain weakly parasitic fungi. Thus, annual cankers usually occur only during the year after unusual weather conditions. Dead tissues eventually slough off annual cankers, and the affected area becomes covered with callus in much the same way a wound is healed. Dieback results when stems and twigs are girdled by annual cankers.

Perennial cankers are caused by biotic agents that remain active in trees for more than 1 year. Sometimes fungi causing perennial cankers kill branches and trees, but more often they weaken and deform the hosts. Usually the circumferential growth of the tree exceeds the growth in canker size, thus preventing the tree from being girdled and killed. Perennial cankers often result in sunken, resinous, unhealed wounds on branches or trunks. Cankers can also be caused by rust fungi and mistletoes (chapters 4 and 5). Perennial cankers caused by other organisms are described in this chapter.

In general, cankers do not constitute a serious disease problem in the coniferous forests of western North America. With few exceptions they seldom reach epidemic proportions. Cankers are considered most serious in plantations and on ornamental or high-value trees. Occasionally, larger trees with trunk cankers constitute a hazard in some high-use areas because they are weakened or decayed at the canker site and may break during high winds.

DESCRIPTIVE KEY

On Monterey cypress .... *Seiridium cardinale*
On redwood .... *Seiridium* sp.
On giant sequoia or incense-cedar .... *Botryosphaeria ribis*
On Douglas-fir
    A^1 Fruiting bodies disc- or cup-shaped when fresh, shriveled when dry .... B
    A^2 Fruiting bodies small, globose, black, mostly embedded in the bark of larger dead branches .... *Diaporthe lokoyae*
    B^1 Center of cup-shaped fruiting body yellow to orange, outer margin hairy .... *Dasyscyphus* sp.
    B^2 Fruiting bodies small (1 to 1.5 mm diameter), black; formed on twigs or branches dead for about 1 year .... *Dermea pseudotsugae*
On true firs
    A^1 No branch dieback, spindle-shaped branch swellings often bearing leafless greenish shoots .... Dwarf mistletoes (chap. 5)
    A^2 Branch dieback resulting in reddish-brown flags .... *Cytospora abietis*
    A^3 Branch and twig dieback but no red-brown flags .... B
    B^1 Dieback of current year's growth only .... *Sclerophoma pythiophila*
    B^2 Dieback on all ages of wood C
    C^1 Fruiting bodies yellow to orange, cup-shaped when fresh or moist, outer surface brown to black, margin hairy (2 to 8 mm diameter) .... *Dasyscyphus* sp.
    C^1 Fruiting bodies black, cup-shaped when fresh or moist ..... D
    D^1 Fruiting bodies small (1 to 2 mm diameter) .... *Cenangium ferruginosum*
    D^2 Fruiting bodies very small (0.5 to 1 mm in diameter) .... *Grovesiella abieticola*

On pines
- A¹ Wood of cankered areas showing blackish stain .... B
- A² Wood of cankered areas not showing blackish stain .... D
- B¹ Sunken trunk cankers common and conspicuous .... *Atropellis piniphila*
- B² Sunken trunk cankers not conspicuous, infection mainly on branches and needles C
- C¹ Noticeable black fruiting bodies, disc-shaped, 1 to 2 mm in diameter on dead or dying branches .... *Atropellis pinicola*
- C² Inconspicuous fruiting bodies, not disc-shaped .... *Sphaeropsis sapinea* or *Sclerophoma pythiophila**
- D¹ Branch swelling often present .... E
- D² Branch swelling not present .... F
- E¹ Small, leafless, orange-green shoots arising from swelling .... dwarf mistletoe (chap. 5)
- E² Spore-bearing, yellow-orange pustules arising from swelling .... rust (chap. 4)
- F¹ Fruiting bodies cup-shaped when moist, yellow or orange, outer margin hairy, 2 to 8 mm diameter ..... *Dasyscyphus* sp.
- F² Fruiting bodies small, globose when fresh or moist, black, 1 to 2 mm in diameter .... *Cenangium ferruginosum*
- F³ Inconspicuous fruiting bodies; abundant pitch exudation on infected twigs, branches, and trunks; reddish, resin-soaked wood; branch and terminal dieback common .... *Fusarium subglutinans*

Atropellis Canker
Atropellis pinicola

Hosts—Sugar pine is the most common host, but western white, ponderosa, and lodgepole pines are also hosts.

Distribution and damage—Although commonly found in western North America, *A. pinicola* mainly infects branches of young, suppressed, and weakened trees and shaded, suppressed, lower branches of larger healthy trees. Except for young sugar pines and western white pines in Oregon and California and lodgepole pines in the Blue Mountains in Oregon, trees seldom are killed or severely damaged. Thus, this fungus poses little threat to vigorous trees in well-managed stands.

Field identification—Typical symptoms and signs of infection by *A. pinicola* include branch flagging, the presence of black fruiting

---

*These two fungi are difficult to differentiate under field conditions and must be examined in the laboratory for positive identification.

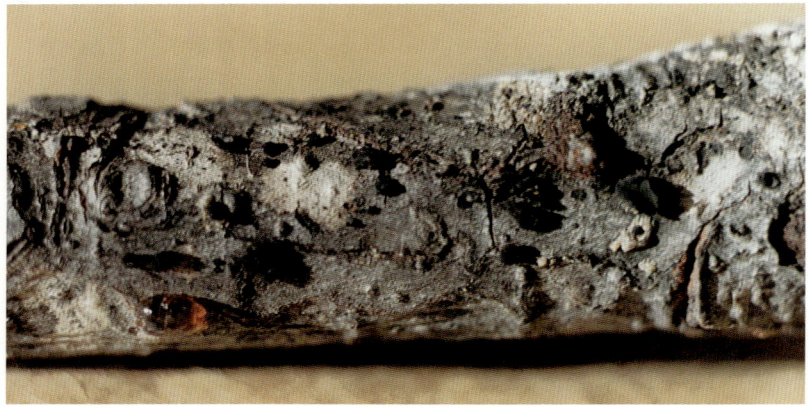

Figure 3-1—*Dried, shriveled, fruiting bodies of* Atropellis pinicola *arising from the bark of a twig of sugar pine.*

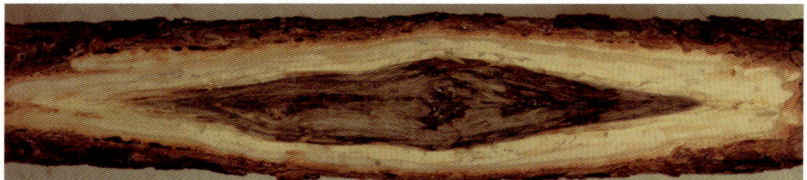

Figure 3-2—*Black stain of the infected wood of a branch of sugar pine infected with* Atropellis pinicola.

bodies 2 to 4 mm in diameter on living or dead branches (fig. 3-1), and a blackish stain of the wood under the dead bark (fig. 3-2). The dry fruiting bodies are shriveled, irregularly shaped structures. Fresh or moist fruiting bodies are cup-shaped.

Atropellis Canker
Atropellis piniphila

Hosts—Lodgepole pine is the only host.

Distribution and damage—*A. piniphila* causes a perennial canker of lodgepole pines in the Pacific Coast States and western Canada. Its southernmost distribution is the northern Sierra Nevada. The organism appears to be restricted in occurrence by rather specific ecologic factors. Infection is often limited to trees growing on cool, moist sites, such as those in wet meadows and around lakeshores. It is also more common in overstocked than in well-spaced stands.

Field identification—The most obvious symptom of infection is the presence of large, sunken, resin-soaked, perennial cankers on the trunks and branches of infected trees (fig. 3-3). Noticeable black, disc-shaped fruiting bodies 2 to 5 mm in size are usually present on the sunken bark surface. A bluish-black stain of the wood at the

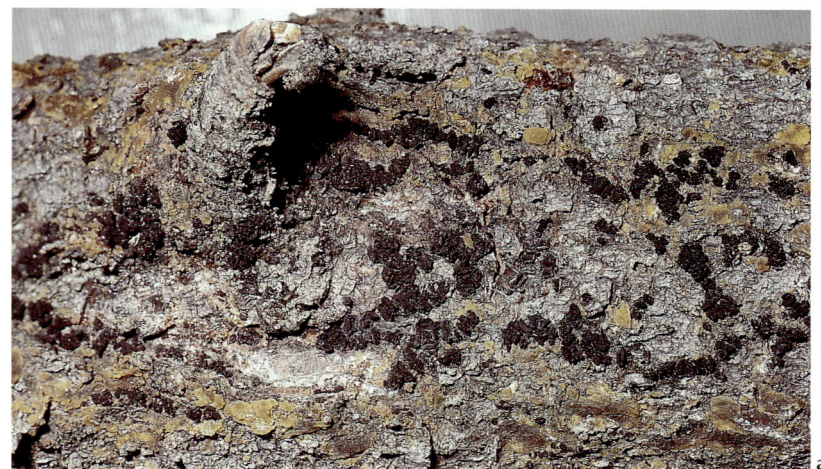

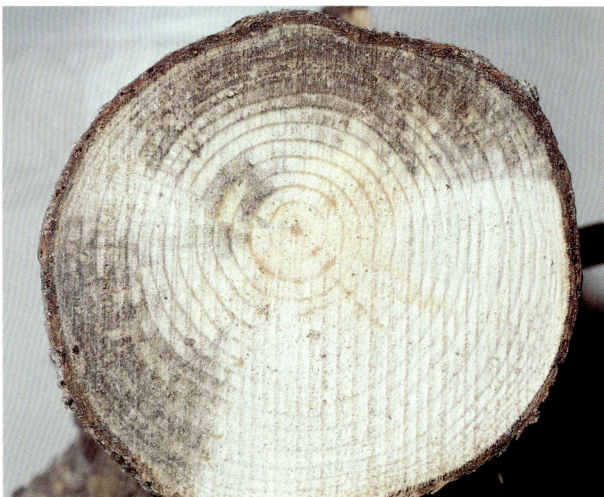

Figure 3-3— Black fruiting bodies protruding from the bark of a lodgepole pine as a result of infection with Atropellis piniphila (**a**). Black stain in the trunk of lodgepole pine infected by A. piniphila (**b**).

canker site is also an apparent symptom for identifying this disease. Although old bole cankers cause severe trunk deformation, only occasionally do they girdle and kill trees. Mortality is most common in small, suppressed trees.

Botryosphaeria Canker
Botryosphaeria ribis

Hosts—Giant sequoia and incense-cedar are the only conifer hosts.

Distribution of damage—*Botryosphaeria* canker is common on giant sequoia and occasionally on incense-cedar planted outside of

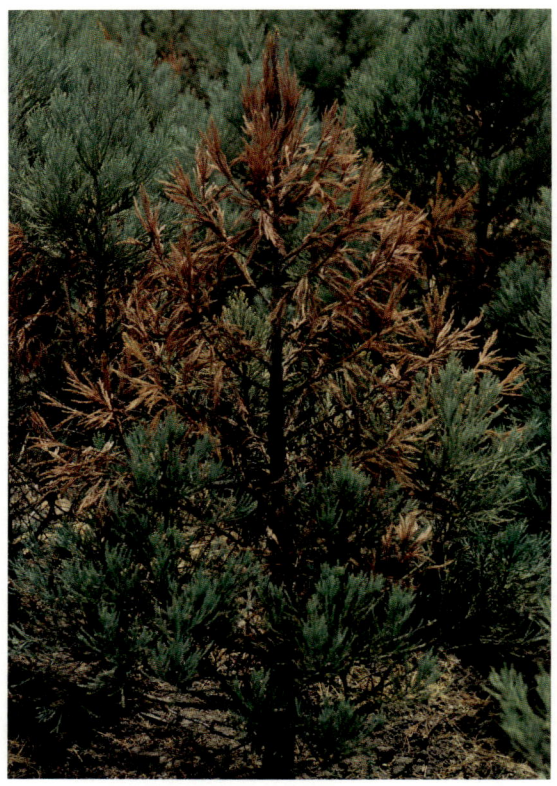

Figure 3-4—*Severe branch flagging of giant sequoia infected by* Botryosphaeria ribis.

the natural range of these species. This organism is particularly damaging when giant sequoia is grown in warmer lower elevational regions in the western United States. Trees in ornamental plantings frequently are attacked after the trees are several years old. The fungus progressively kills branches and may severely damage or kill trees.

Field identification—Initial symptoms of infection are scattered dieback of twigs and branches. With time, the fungus builds up and spreads throughout the crown, occasionally killing the tops. Recently killed branches appear as reddish-brown flags (fig. 3-4); branches dead for longer periods are gray-brown and bare of much of their foliage. Infected branches often exude drops of pitch.

Cenangium Canker
Cenangium ferruginosum

Hosts—Jeffrey pine is the common host, but *Cenangium* canker also occurs on other pines and true firs.

Distribution and damage—This organism occurs throughout western North America, most commonly on trees up to pole size. It is

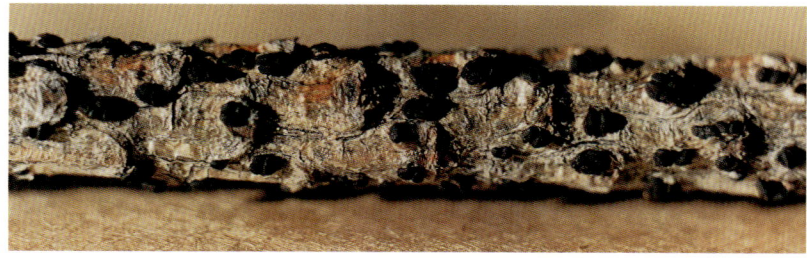

Figure 3-5—*Clustered black fruiting bodies of* Cenangium ferruginosum, *arising from within the bark of a branch of Jeffrey pine.*

a weak parasite and seldom kills trees. Suppressed or weakened lower branches are most commonly infected, but trees growing under poor conditions or weakened from other causes may be more severely attacked.

Field identification—Symptoms and signs of *Cenangium* infection include dead or dying lower branches usually 2 cm or less in diameter and small, black fruiting bodies 1 to 2 mm in diameter on the dead branches. The fruiting bodies are cup-shaped when fresh or moist and shriveled when dry (fig. 3-5). No black stain of the infected wood is associated with this fungus, unlike *Atropellis pinicola.*

Cytospora Canker of True Firs
Cytospora abietis

Hosts—True firs are the most common hosts. Douglas-fir is rarely infected.

Distribution and damage—*Cytospora abietis* is a damaging, canker-inducing fungus that commonly occurs on true firs throughout their natural range in California, central and eastern Oregon, and frequently on firs and Douglas-fir elsewhere in the western United States. A weak parasite, it attacks only trees that have been debilitated by other disease-causing agents, drought, fire, insects, and human activities.

One of the important factors that predisposes firs to attack by *C. abietis* is dwarf mistletoe (*Arceuthobium*). Practically all fir stands in California and Oregon infested with dwarf mistletoe are attacked by this fungus. *C. abietis* more commonly infects branches invaded by dwarf mistletoe; in some stands, nearly a fourth of all branches bearing mistletoe are infected. Thus, in mistletoe-infested fir stands, considerable branch killing occurs each year as a result of this canker organism. Because this fungus is widely found in true fir stands and occasionally reaches damaging proportions in certain years, *C. abietis* can constitute a threat to the management of these tree species.

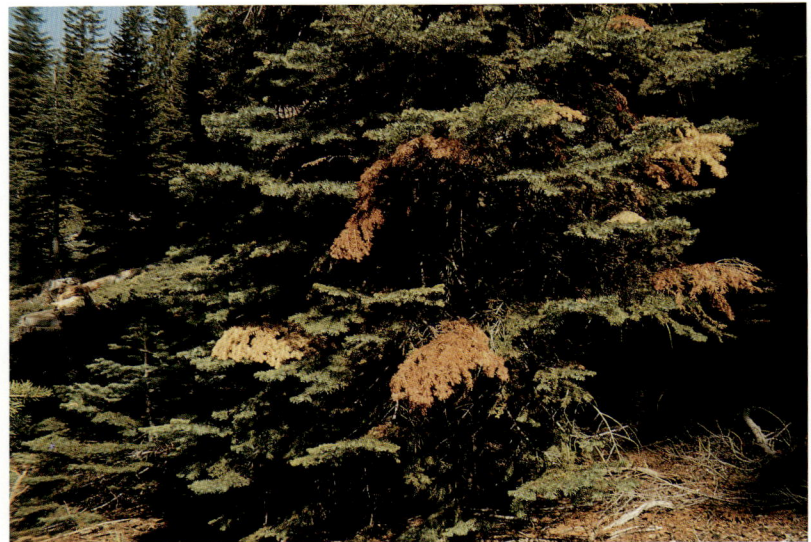

Figure 3-6—*Branch flagging of red fir caused by* Cytospora abietis.

Field identification—Numerous brick-red flagged branches, conspicuous in spring and summer, are the best symptoms of the disease (fig. 3-6). Later in the year the foliage dries and becomes more brown to tan in appearance. Trees of all ages are attacked. Young trees or tops of young trees are often killed by the fungus, whereas only branches are killed on larger trees. Other symptoms and signs of infection are sunken, dead patches of bark tissue, resin exudation at the canker site, small pimple-like fruiting bodies embedded in the dead bark, and thread-like spore masses exuded from the fruiting bodies (fig. 3-7).

Dasyscyphus Canker of Conifers
Dasyscyphus spp.

Hosts—Common hosts include Douglas-fir, pines, and true firs.

Distribution and damage—Apparently, more than one fungus species is involved, and these attack several conifer species in western North America. The disease is spotty in occurrence and seldom causes serious damage. It appears to be most serious on Douglas-fir and on pines growing at high-elevations. Otherwise, *Dasyscyphus* species are weak parasites and infect only weakened or suppressed lower branches and twigs. Occasionally, trunk cankers may develop on small trees.

Field identification—The fruiting bodies of the fungus are quite distinctive. When fresh or moist, they are cup-shaped, vary in color from a light cream to orange, have a fuzzy outer margin, and are about 2 to 8 mm in diameter (fig. 3-8). When dry, they appear as shriveled light-colored bodies on the dead bark of the infected branch or canker.

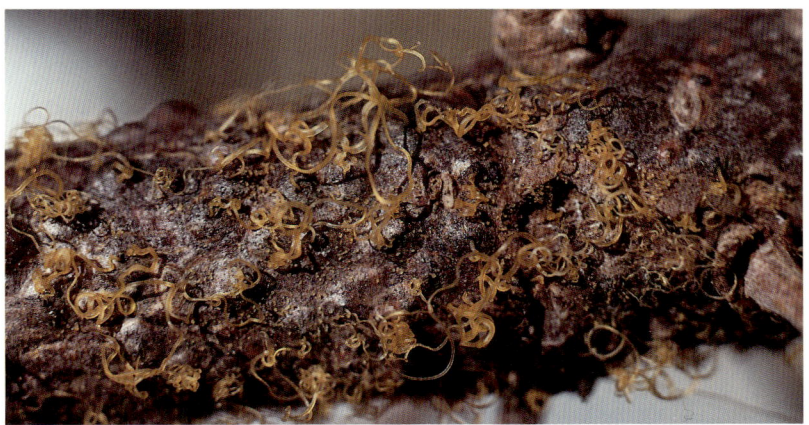

Figure 3-7—*Orange thread-like spore masses exuded from the fruiting bodies of* Cytospora abietis *partially embedded within the bark of red fir.*

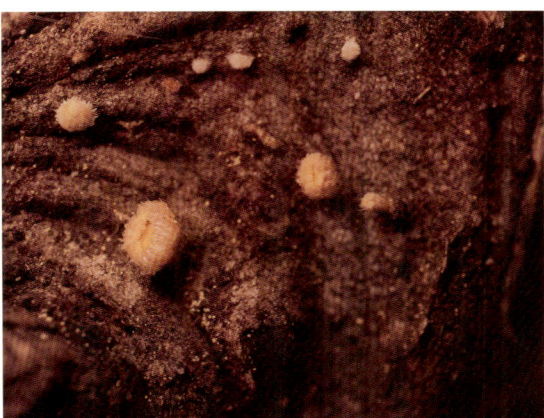

Figure 3-8—*Orange, cup-shaped fruiting bodies formed on branches of white fir infected by the fungus,* Dasyscyphus sp.

The wood of the infected branch at the canker site does not stain black as it does with some of the other canker fungi.

Dermea Canker
Dermea pseudotsugae

Hosts—Douglas-fir and occasionally grand fir are the common hosts.

Distribution and damage—This canker severely damages Douglas-fir and to a lesser extent grand fir from northwestern California to British Columbia. Plantations of young trees are most often attacked, but the fungus also develops on young trees in natural stands. In some plantations surveyed, 10 to 50 percent of the trees were killed by this organism in less than 10 years. Both limb dieback and trunk cankers occur on infected trees. Trunk cankers often girdle the tree, resulting in top kill and eventual death of the tree. Frosts or periods of below-normal precipitation are known to predispose trees to infection.

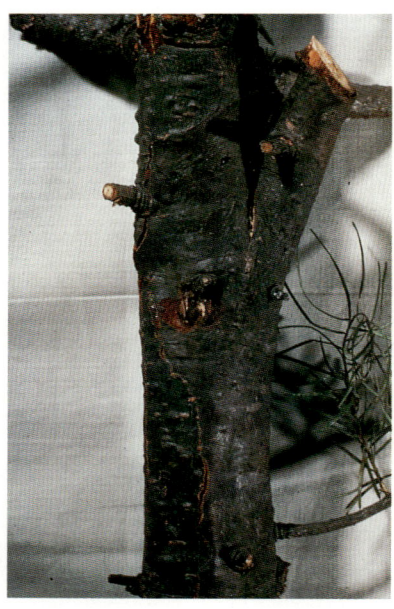

Figure 3-9—*Dermea canker caused by* Dermea pseudotsugae *on the trunk of a sapling-sized Douglas-fir.*

Field identification—Dieback of limbs, tops, and entire trees is the most obvious symptom of the disease. Trunk cankers originate from infected limbs and when fresh have a characteristic reddish margin that disappears when the tree dies (fig. 3-9). Sexual fruiting bodies (apothecia) do not appear on freshly killed tissue but arise on dead bark about a year later. They appear as tiny, black discs about 1.0 to 1.5 mm in diameter. The Douglas-fir engraver, *Scolytus unispinosus*, is often associated with cankers.

Phomopsis Canker of Douglas-fir
Diaporthe (Phomopsis) lokoyae

Hosts—Douglas-fir is the known host.

Distribution and damage—*Phomopsis* canker of Douglas-fir is most common in the northern part of the Coast Range of California and southeast Oregon but can be found in other natural and planted stands elsewhere along the Pacific Coast. It occurs sporadically and becomes a problem only during years of drought stress or when similar climatic conditions weaken the host and favor buildup of the fungus. Usually only single trees or small groups of trees are affected. The disease is primarily one of young trees. Trees up to 3 inches (8 cm) in diameter are often killed by the fungus whereas larger ones usually survive. On larger trees, tops and branches are often killed. Cankers may also develop on the trunk. After the initial attack, cankers often heal in much the same way an axe wound heals. The fungus, for the most part, is not a serious problem in natural forest stands but in nurseries, forest plantations, and Christmas tree farms, it occasionally causes serious damage and economic loss.

Field identification—Branch or trunk cankers are the best symptom of the disease. Cankers almost always result when the fungus first infects young twigs and branches and then grows into the adjoining stem. Cankers are usually sunken and several times longer than they are wide (fig. 3-10). On branches and tree tops girdled by the fungus

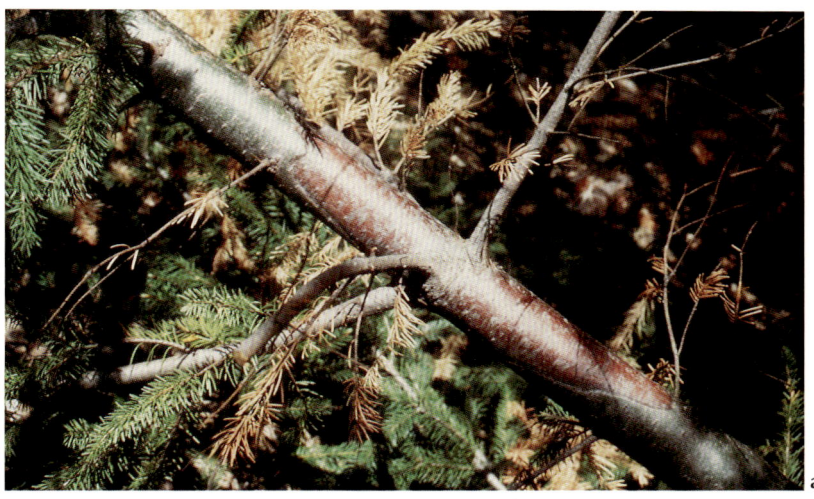

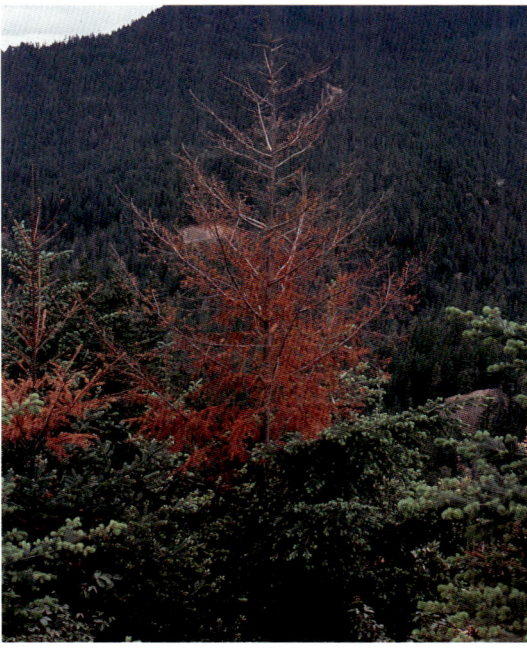

Figure 3-10—*Phomopsis canker of a young Douglas-fir resulting from infection by Diaporthe (*Phomopsis*) lokoyae* (***a***). *Tops of Douglas-fir can be girdled and killed by* Diaporthe lokoyae (***b***).

Figure 3-11—*Scattered, dying branches on Monterey pine infected by Fusarium subglutinans, the cause of pine pitch canker.*

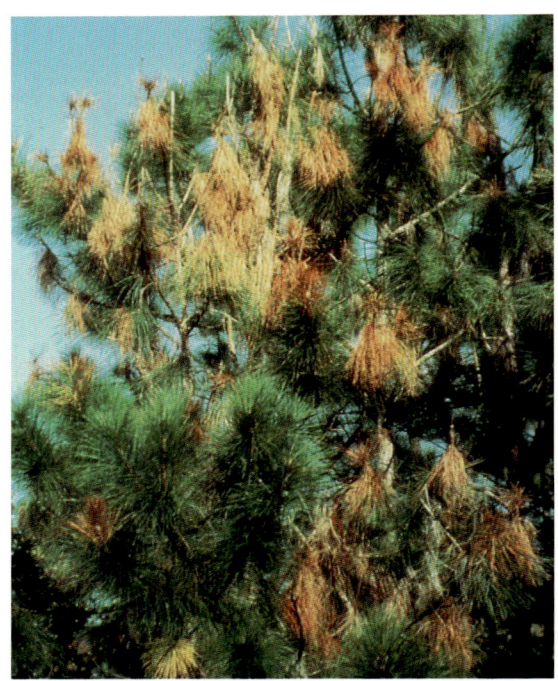

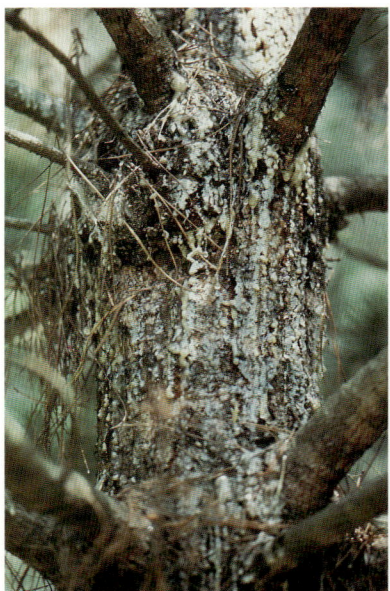

Figure 3-12—*Abundant resin flow from infected branches and trunks is an obvious symptom of pitch canker of pines.*

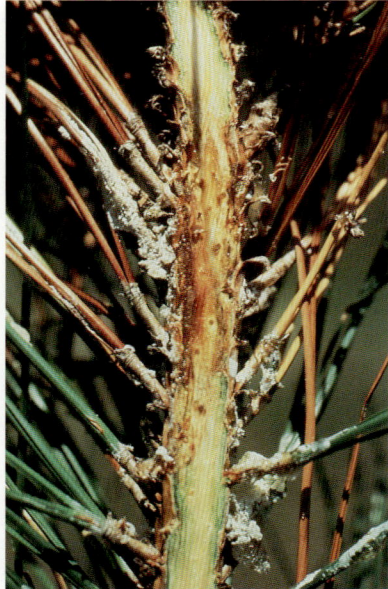

Figure 3-13—*Pitch-infiltrated dying shoot of Monterey pine infected with pine pitch canker.*

there is usually a distinct margin between the infected and the healthy portions of the stems. Small, black fruiting bodies (less than 0.5 mm diameter) embedded in the dead bark may be seen in spring and early summer on the cankered tissues. Phomopsis cankers are similar to those caused by *Dermea pseudotsugae* but have no conspicuous reddish margin.

Pitch Canker of Pines
Fusarium subglutinans

Hosts—The fungus has been found in the field on Monterey, Bishop, Aleppo, and Italian stone pines. (Most western pines tested in the greenhouse are susceptible to the pitch canker fungus.)

Distribution and damage—Pitch canker was first found on Monterey pines in Santa Cruz County, CA, in summer 1986. Subsequent surveys indicated that several thousand trees were infected. Counties with fewer diseased trees include Monterey, Alameda, Santa Barbara, Los Angeles, San Diego, Santa Clara, San Mateo, and San Luis Obispo. The disease has been known for decades to be a problem on pines in the southeastern United States and has recently been reported in several pine stands in Mexico. The disease can be very damaging to susceptible pines of all sizes. It has been found in mature planted trees, Christmas tree plantations, and nurseries. It has not been reported in native forest stands in California. Conspicuous branch flagging, top kill, and tree death (particularly in small trees and seedlings) are obvious symptoms of pitch canker.

Disease cycle—The fungus spreads by means of spores produced in small pink fruiting bodies called sporodochia. Sporodochia are produced mostly on infected branches, twigs, and cones. Spore production, spread, and infection most likely occur during periods of rain. Wounds are required for infection, and some insects are known to carry and transmit the disease. The disease is known to be seedborne and can spread to other areas on contaminated seed and young seedlings. Some trees within areas of heavy infection have shown strong resistance to the disease.

Field identification—Branch flagging and top kill are the most obvious symptoms of the disease (fig. 3-11). Abundant resin flow from branch and trunk cankers is also an obvious symptom (fig. 3-12). Another obvious symptom is heavy resin soaking of the wood of infected branches and trunks (fig. 3-13). Fruiting bodies may or may not be present on the diseased tree parts; when present they appear most often on the younger portions of dead tissue. For positive diagnosis of the disease, tissue needs to be taken to the laboratory for culturing and identification of the fungus.

Diplodia Canker
Sphaeropsis sapinea (Diplodia pinea)

Hosts—This fungus infects pines, rarely Douglas-fir.

Distribution and damage—This fungus may occur on pines throughout the western United States. In California it is found on low-elevation and coastal pine species. The fungus is a weak parasite and usually infects only trees that are planted out of their natural environment or are weakened by drought or other agents. For example, branches weakened by dwarf mistletoe infection are reported to be commonly attacked and killed by this organism. The fungus spreads from infected branches into the trunks of trees, causing top kill or tree mortality. For the most part, however, vigorous trees suffer only dieback of weakened branches as a result of infection by *S. sapinea*.

Disease cycle—This fungus is one of the few canker- and dieback-inducing organisms that also infects needles. Infection takes place through the stomata of young needles. The fungus then grows through the needles into young twigs, causing a dieback. Infection by spores may also occur through wounds or bark cracks on branches. Much of the dieback and cankering of older branches and trunks probably takes place this way.

Field identification—Dying needles and twigs as well as top dieback and tree mortality are indicative of infection by *S. sapinea*. The fruiting bodies are small (less than 0.5 mm in diameter), black, globose, and embedded within the needles or bark of infected stems. Usually only the beak of the fruiting body protrudes through the surface of the infected tissues, and these beaks resemble numerous small, black pinpoint spots. A noticeable black stain of the wood is also associated with infection by *S. sapinea*.

Sclerophoma Canker of Pines
Sclerophoma pythiophila

Hosts—The known hosts are pines.

Distribution and damage—This fungus is known to be a weak parasite of pines. It grows mostly on smaller trees up to about 15 to 20 feet (4.6 to 6.1 m) in height. The disease causes no threat to forest stands but may damage trees in plantations or trees grown for ornamental purposes.

Field identification—This fungus causes mainly a twig disease although branches may occasionally be defoliated. Trees may suffer from top dieback and occasionally are killed back two or three whorls. Infected wood is stained a bluish black. Symptoms and signs in the field closely resemble those caused by *Sphaeropsis sapinea*. Laboratory examination is often necessary to distinguish between these two fungi.

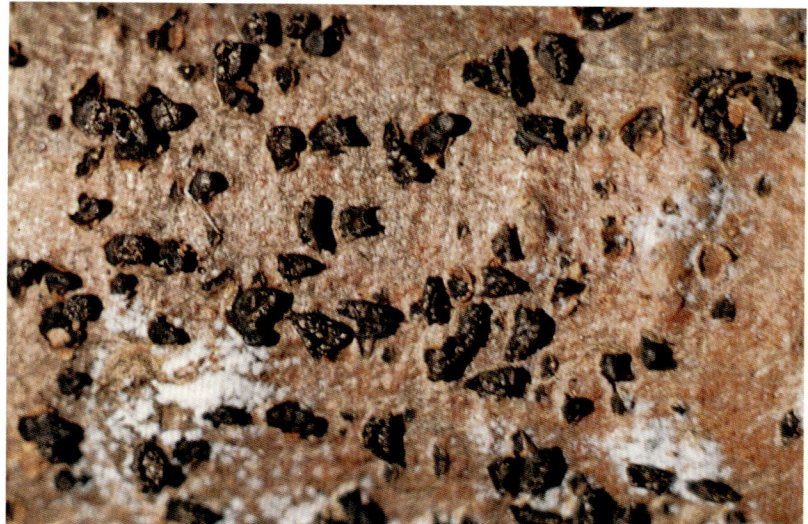

Figure 3-14—*Scattered, small, black fruiting bodies on the surface of a branch of white fir infected by the canker fungus* Grovesiella abieticola.

Grovesiella Canker
Grovesiella abieticola (Scleroderris abieticola)

Hosts—Hosts include white fir, grand fir, Pacific silver fir, subalpine fir, and California red fir.

Distribution and damage—This fungus grows on *Abies* along the Pacific Coast from northern California through British Columbia. Highly sporadic in occurrence, it is usually not a serious disease-causing agent. Annual cankers and twig dieback develop as a result of infection, and these conditions usually do not continue for more than 1 year. Occasionally some tops are killed. Small trees are most often attacked, but lower branches of poles sometimes are infected.

Field identification—The fruiting bodies of this fungus are similar to but somewhat smaller (0.5 to 1 mm in diameter) than the black, cup-shaped fruiting bodies of *Cenangium* that are also found on firs. The fruiting bodies of *G. abieticola*, although small, are usually very abundant on the dead bark (fig. 3-14). This organism is seldom found on 1-year-old wood but does attack older stems. Canker development is often pronounced, but no staining of wood accompanies infection.

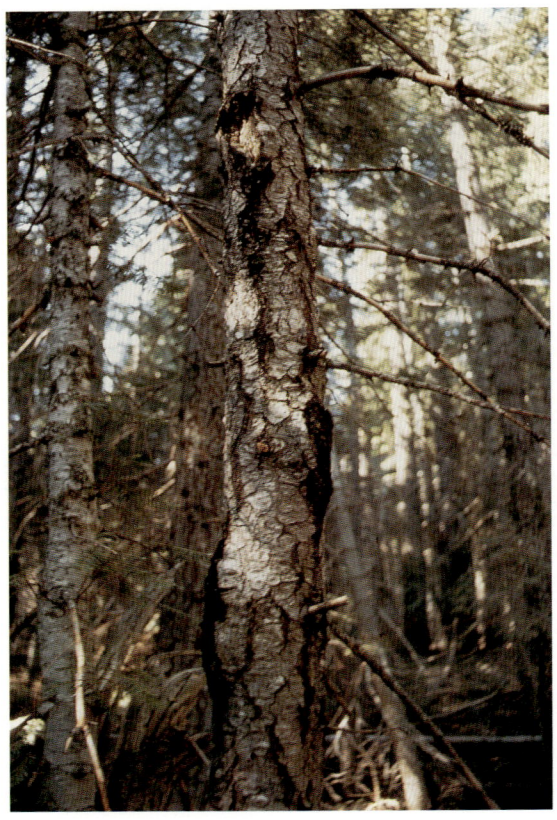

Figure 3-15—*A large, open canker caused by* Nectria fuckeliana *has developed on the lower trunk of a white fir.*

Nectria Canker of White Fir
Nectria fuckeliana

Hosts—The known host is white fir.

Distribution and damage—*Nectria* canker was first reported on white firs in northern California in 1978. Subsequent investigations showed that the range of the disease extended from northern California into southern Oregon. Damage consists mainly of trunk deformation and tree death due to breakage at the canker site.

Disease cycle—Little is known about the disease cycle. The disease is found most often in stands with large numbers of small trees and where white fir is the major stand component. Infection is possibly through wounds or injuries caused by insects.

Field identification—Conspicuous trunk cankers are the most obvious symptom of *Nectria* canker (fig. 3-15). Most cankers occur on small, suppressed trees less than 6 inches (15 cm) dbh. Fruiting bodies, when present, usually are found around the canker margins (fig. 3-16) and are more common on dead rather than live trees.

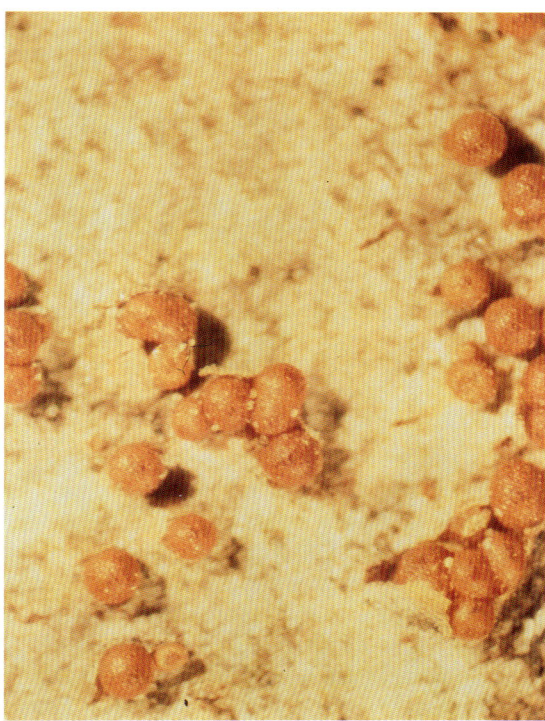

Figure 3-16—*Orange, round fruiting bodies about 1 to 2 mm in diameter of* Nectria fuckeliana *are produced at the margins of developed cankers.*

Certain lepidopteran insects (Noctuidae) are often associated with the canker and apparently prevent host callus formation and containment of the fungus.

Cypress Canker
Seiridium cardinale (Coryneum cardinale)

Hosts—Principal host of this canker is Monterey cypress; occasional hosts are other species of cypress, but rarely juniper.

Distribution and damage—Cypress canker is absent from native stands of Monterey cypress and is rare on planted cypress immediately along the Pacific Coast. However, the disease is widespread and serious on Monterey cypress planted in the warmer, drier inland areas. Over the period of about a decade in the early 1900's, the fungus spread throughout the range of planted Monterey cypress in the western United States.

The branch flagging and tree death caused by this organism was so severe that planting Monterey cypress outside of its natural range is discouraged. Why the fungus suddenly appeared and became epidemic on planted Monterey cypress is not known, but it is now widespread and well established.

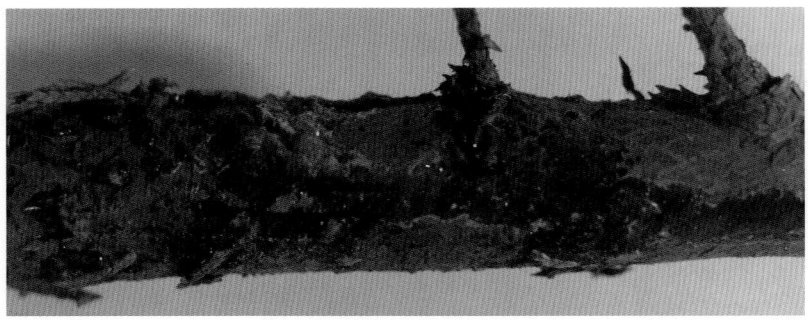

Figure 3-17—*Branch of Monterey cypress infected by the cypress canker fungus (Seiridium cardinale). Note abundant resin flow and small, black fruiting bodies on bark surface.*

Infection cycle—Cypress canker is spread over long distances by windblown spores; locally and within tree crowns, it is spread by spores washed out of the fruiting bodies by rains. Most infections occur at the bases of small branches or in branch forks. Both wounded and unwounded tissues are sites of infection.

Cankers grow more rapidly along a branch than around it, and they usually have a length-width ratio of about 3 to 1. Infected trees or branches 2 to 3 years old may be killed within a year, whereas infected branches or trunks of larger trees may remain alive for 5 to 10 years.

Field identification—Fading and death of twigs, branches, and tops of trees are the most conspicuous symptoms of infection. Trees of all ages and sizes are equally susceptible to infection. The presence of cankers (fig. 3-17) is a sure indication of infection. Resin flow usually accompanies canker development, and as the killed bark tissues dry out, a sunken area develops. Bark cracking commonly accompanies canker development. Dark, irregularly shaped, blister-like fruiting bodies 0.3 to 1.5 mm in size are produced and break through the bark of the dead tissues. Cypress bark beetles are often associated with, and hasten the death of, infected trees.

Redwood Canker
Seiridium sp.

Hosts—Coast redwood is the only known host.

Distribution and damage—Redwood canker is found in native stands of redwood north of San Francisco. For the most part, it occurs only spottily and appears to be most common on redwood trees on poor sites. For example, trees growing on warm, dry southern slopes in Mendocino County have occasionally suffered severe branch dieback and top kill (fig. 3-18). Smaller trees are most commonly infected and usually the lower branches are attacked first. However,

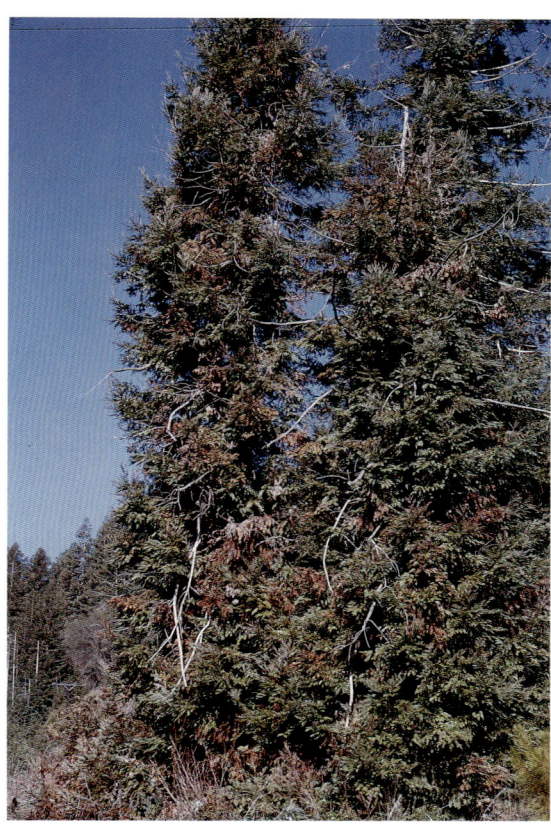

Figure 3-18— *Branch flagging of coast redwood caused by the redwood canker fungus (Seiridium sp).*

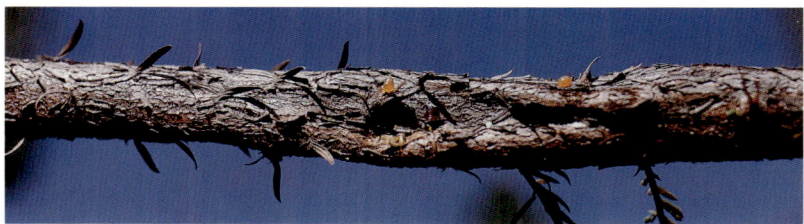

Figure 3-19— *Sunken branch cankers often result from infection of coast redwood by Seiridium sp.*

this fungus has been observed killing branches in the tops of old-growth redwood. Sunken, resinous branch cankers are common on infected branches (fig. 3-19).

Field identification—Symptoms of this disease are nearly identical to symptoms of the cypress canker in Monterey cypress. In fact, there is some evidence that the redwood canker fungus and the cypress canker fungus may be the same species. Further studies are needed, however, to determine the differences in taxonomy and host-disease relationships of these two canker fungi.

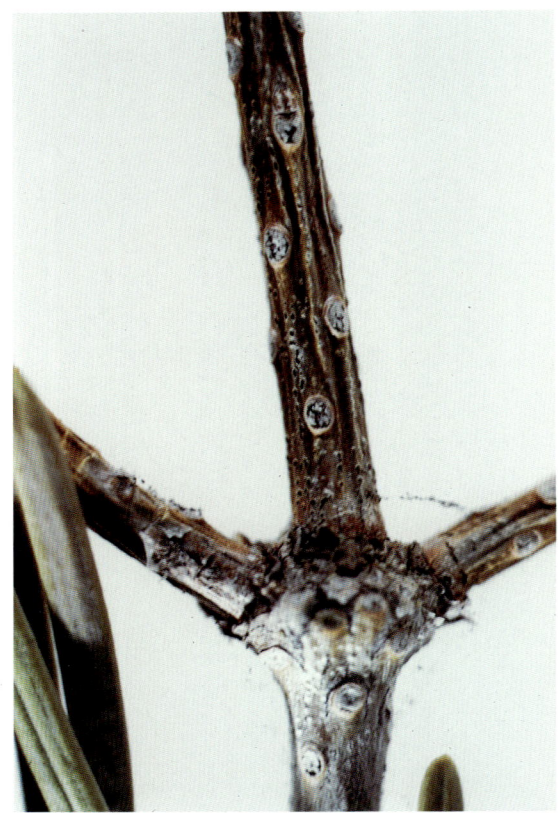

Figure 3-20— *Sclerophoma* tip dieback of white fir caused by Sclerophoma pythiophila. Note the small, black fruiting bodies on the dead twig.

Sclerophoma Tip Dieback of Fir
Sclerophoma pythiophila (Sydowia polyspora)

Hosts—The hosts are pines, Douglas-fir, true firs, spruce, hemlock, larch, and arborvitae.

Distribution and damage—*Sclerophoma pythiophila* has been reported on many conifers along the Pacific Coast. In California it is a problem primarily in white fir stands managed for Christmas trees. From the timber management standpoint, damage is negligible. In general, infection results in branch cankers and tip dieback after frost damage, injury, or drought.

Field identification—The symptoms and signs of sclerophoma tip dieback closely resemble those of grovesiella canker. But *S. pythiophila* infects only 1-year-old wood, causing tip dieback (fig. 3-20). Occasionally, a canker margin may be found about a third of the way down 2-year-old wood on a branch. Black fruiting bodies less than 0.2 mm in diameter appear from under the bark of twigs that have been dead for a year or more.

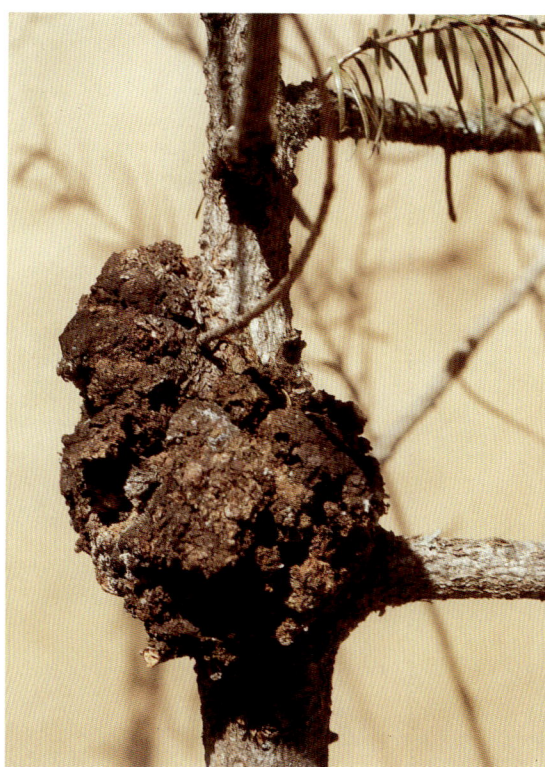

Figure 3-21—
Bacterial gall of Douglas-fir caused by Pseudomonas pseudotsugae.

GALLS

Many galls found in conifers in California are of unknown origin, but some are caused by bacteria, insects, rust fungi, and mistletoes. Although numerous on some hosts in certain areas, galls are relatively unimportant forest diseases. They are usually found on scattered trees rather than on most trees in a stand. They cause relatively little damage to the trees on which they develop—except for galls that occasionally occur on the main stem.

Gall of Douglas-fir

A gall of Douglas-fir has been reported to be caused by the bacterium *Pseudomonas pseudotsugae*; however, recent efforts by plant pathologists at the University of California, Berkeley, failed to confirm this report. Repeated efforts to isolate a bacterial pathogen have failed. Therefore, the cause of these galls on Douglas-fir is unknown. The galls are commonly observed on young Douglas-fir in northern California and Oregon. Galls are roughly globose and may become several inches in diameter (fig. 3-21). Tops of young trees may be killed, but galls on branches or boles of larger trees affect growth only slightly.

Galls of Unknown Origin

Redwood gall, a gall of unknown origin, develops on coast redwood. Often huge galls grow on the trunks of old-growth redwood. Because of their beautifully figured grain, they are highly prized for use in furniture or for novelty items. Galls also occur on branches. Occasional trees support many of them with little apparent effect on growth or vigor of the tree.

Other galls of unknown origin also are found on other conifers, particularly the pines, in the western United States. Their effect on the growth of trees is minimal. They are of no real importance in the management of forest lands. Galls caused by rust fungi and mistletoes are covered in chapters 5 and 6.

SELECTED REFERENCES

Bega, Robert V. 1964. Diseases of sequoia. Diseases of widely planted forest trees. FAO/IUFRO Symposium on internationally dangerous forest diseases and insects; 1964 July 20–30; Oxford, England. Washington, DC: U.S. Department of Agriculture, Forest Service: 131–139.

Boyce, John S. 1933. A canker of Douglas-fir associated with *Phomopsis lokoyae*. Journal of Forestry 31:664–672.

Funk, A. 1967. *Dermea pseudotsugae* n. sp., a causal agent of phloem necrosis in Douglas-fir. Canadian Journal of Botany 15:1803–1809.

Funk, A. 1973. *Phomopsis (Diaporthe)* canker of Douglas-fir in British Columbia. For. Insect Dis. Surv. Pest Leafl. 60. Victoria, BC: Canadian Forestry Service.

Funk, A. 1981. Parasitic microfungi of western trees. CC-X-222. Victoria, BC: Canadian Forestry Research Centre.

Hansen, H.N.; Smith, R.E. 1937. A bacterial gall disease of Douglas-fir, *Pseudotsugae taxifolia*. Hilgardia 10:569–577.

Lightle, Paul C.; Thompson, J.H. 1973. *Atropellis* canker of pines. For. Pest Leafl. 138. Washington, DC: U.S. Department of Agriculture, Forest Service. 6 p.

McCain, Arthur H.; Koehler, Carlton S.; Tjosvold, Steven A. 1987. Pitch canker threatens California pines. California Agriculture November-December, p. 22–23.

Scharpf, Robert F. 1969. *Cytospora abietis* associated with dwarf mistletoe on true firs in California. Phytopathology 59:1657–1658.

Schultz, Mark E.; Parmeter, John R., Jr. 1990. A canker disease of *Abies concolor* caused by *Nectria fuckeliana*. Plant Disease 74:178–180.

Sutton, B.C. 1980. The Coeiomycetes. Kew, Surrey, England: Commonwealth Mycological Institute. 696 p.

Sutton, B.C.; Gibson, I.A.S. 1972. *Seiridium cardinale*: descriptions of pathogenic fungi and bacteria. No. 326. Kew, Surrey, England: Commonwealth Mycological Institute. 2 p.

Wagener, Willis W. 1939. The canker of Cupressus induced by *Coryneum cardinale* n. sp. Journal of Agricultural Research 58:1–46.

Wright, Ernest. 1942. *Cytospora abietis*: the cause of a canker of true firs in California and Nevada. Journal of Agricultural Research 65:113–153.

CHAPTER 4   Rusts

Robert V. Bega and Robert F. Scharpf

Robert V. Bega (retired) was in charge of the Pacific Southwest Research Station's research unit investigating the biology and control of diseases of conifer forests, headquartered in Albany, CA.

Robert F. Scharpf, Scientist Emeritus, was Project Leader, Disease Research and Principal Plant Pathologist, Pacific Southwest Research Station, Forest Service, U.S. Department of Agriculture, Albany, CA.

INTRODUCTION

Rust diseases are caused by fungi that are obligate parasites, that is, fungi that develop only on living hosts. Most rusts described in this chapter are considered **native rusts**. Native rusts are often widespread but cause less damage to their hosts than some of the introduced rusts like *Cronartium ribicola*. Nonetheless, native rusts kill individual trees, reduce wood quality, and retard tree growth. More than 50 species of native rust fungi are known to attack conifers in the western United States, but only a few cause important diseases of western conifers. To complete their life cycles, nearly all the major rust fungi on conifers must alternate between the conifer host and an unrelated type of host plant. Those that require two different hosts are called **heteroecious rusts**. Most produce four to five different kinds of spore stages, as indicated either by name or by roman numerals (0 through IV) (figure 4-1). Two major rust diseases—western gall rust and a limb rust—do not need to alternate between unrelated host plants but spread directly. Such rusts, which do not require an alternate host, are called **autoecious rusts**.

Pycnia (0) are the first spore bodies produced on the **aecial host**. **Pycniospores,** which serve in sexual fertilization, are exuded from the pycnia and are not known to be infective agents. Sexual fertilization is required before maturation of the **aecial stage** (I), which produces **aeciospores,** which can infect the alternate host, sometimes as far as 600 to 800 miles (966 to 1,287 km) distant from their point source. On the alternate hosts rusts of most genera produce the repeating or **uredial stage** (II) from which **urediospores** are produced. These, again, are dispersed short distances by wind and infect other individuals of the same host species or reinfect the plant on which they were borne. Later, these infections produce the **telial stage** (III), which is composed of **teliospores**, which remain in place and germinate under the right climatic conditions in a few days to produce **basidiospores** (also called **sporidia**) (IV). Windborne for short distances, basidiospores infect only the aecial host.

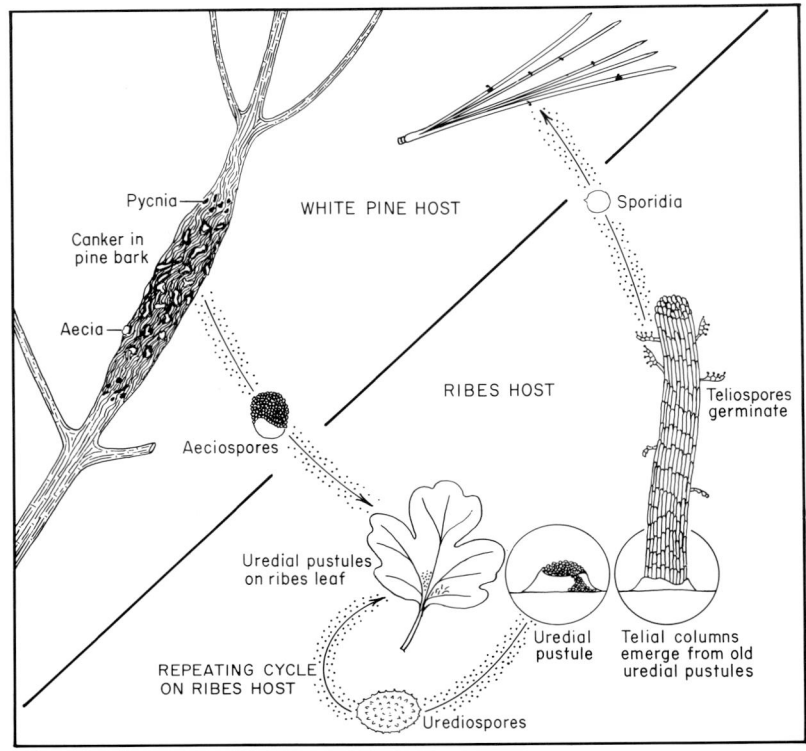

Figure 4-1—*Life cycle of white pine blister rust (Cronartium ribicola).*

Local climate and land uses that favor growth of alternate hosts often intensify rust diseases. For example, *Ribes* species must be closely associated with pinyon in a favorable regime of moisture and temperature before infection of pines by pinyon rust *(Cronartium occidentale)* can occur. Similarly, concentrations of *Comandra* species are needed to trigger outbreaks of comandra rust *(C. comandrae).* Western gall rust *(Peridermium harknessii),* an autoecious rust, will be most troublesome in localities where high humidity and moderately cool temperatures prevail or where there are even-aged young stands or plantations. This gall rust can be especially destructive in nurseries and ornamental plantings.

An intricately balanced interaction of host, parasite, and environmental factors determines rust outbreaks. Most outbreaks involve a burst of infection during a single season or even a single moist period, and then years may pass with no new infections occurring. Major outbreaks may come decades apart. Even with the fungus *P. harknessii,* which spreads from pine to pine, infection may be sporadic in spite of its simplified life cycle. Among the numerous rust fungi that attack conifers, most are minor needle rusts that cause partial defoliation only during years favorable for infection. Some rusts may be more damaging to their alternate hosts. Several native rusts cause deformities, dieback, and limited mortality to conifers of little commercial value but of high recreational and esthetic value. The most damaging rusts in the western United States are white pine blister rust on white pines; comandra rust, western gall rust, stalactiform canker rust, and filamentosum limb rust on hard pines; broom rust on true firs and spruce; and broom rust on incense-cedar. Others are a problem only in selected areas, such as Christmas tree farms and recreational sites.

RUSTS ON PINES

White Pine Blister Rust
Cronartium ribicola

White pine blister rust, caused by the rust fungus *Cronartium ribicola,* is a textbook example of a heteroecious rust fungus. Its life cycle, symptoms, and climatic requirements are typical of most native western rust fungi described in this chapter. It differs only in its rate of spread and the amount of damage that it causes.

Hosts—*C. ribicola* can infect nearly all white pines and is restricted to this group. Its native North American hosts are eastern white pine, western white pine, sugar pine, limber pine, whitebark pine, bristlecone pine, foxtail pine, and Mexican white pine. In addition, it infects all species of the genus *Ribes*, its alternate host.

Distribution and damage—The disease was introduced into North America in the early 1900's on seedlings of eastern white pine grown in Europe. It was not native to Europe, however, but is believed to have been introduced into that continent from Asia. Its introduction to North America resulted in one of our most serious disease outbreaks on conifers. White pine blister rust is now widely found in northeastern United States, the Lake States, and the West. It was introduced into British Columbia in 1910 and has spread from there throughout most white pine regions of Washington, Idaho, Montana, Wyoming, Oregon, and California.

In North America, white pine blister rust has caused more damage and costs more to control than any other conifer disease. Since the 1920's, millions of dollars have been spent on the eradication of the alternate host, *Ribes*, and thousands of white pine stands have been severely damaged. In the western United States and Canada, some stands have been completely destroyed. When the main stem of a tree is invaded, death is only a question of time. Frequently, in western white pine and sugar pine, death results without trunk infection—the branches are killed by numerous infections before the disease reaches the main stem.

Figure 4-2—*Aecial state of white pine blister rust on sugar pine.*

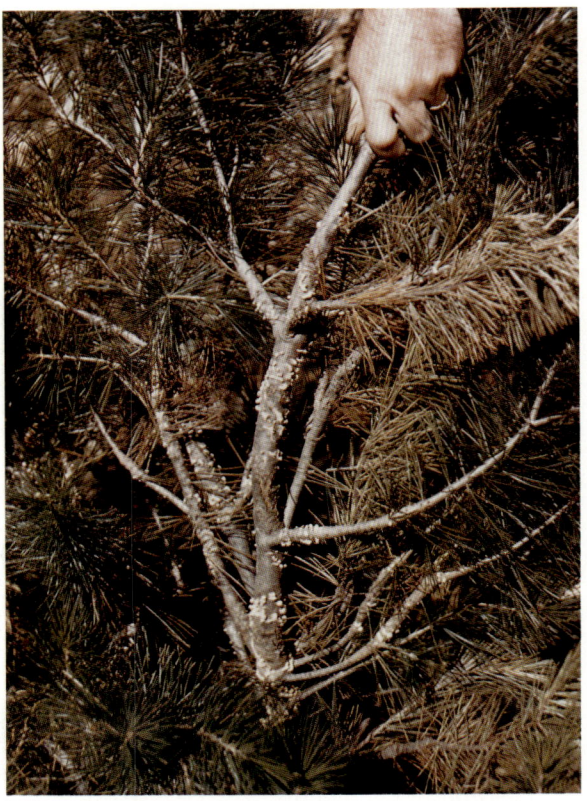

Disease cycle—The sporidia produced from the teliospores on leaves of *Ribes* species are windblown for short distances and infect pine needles during late summer and early autumn. Infection can take place on needles of the current year but is more frequent on 2- to 3-year-old needles. One to two, frequently three years after infection, the fungus has penetrated the needle into the stem and becomes obvious as a yellow or orange discoloration of the bark accompanied by a spindle-shaped swelling. Later pycnia appear as small blisters on the bark. These blisters then discharge droplets of honey-colored liquid containing pycniospores, which are thought to play a sexual role and are required for the production of the aecial stage. Aecia produced from aeciospores are the prominent blisters (fig. 4-2) that burst in spring to disclose masses of orange spores.

Aeciospores can travel long distances—as much as 600 to 800 miles (966 to 1,287 km)—to infect young *Ribes* leaves. Within a few weeks of infection, small yellow uredial pustules appear on the lower leaf surfaces. The resultant urediospores infect other *Ribes* but cannot infect pines. This stage of the fungus is the **repeating stage**. The spores are airborne for only short distances and infect not only other species of *Ribes*, but also can intensify on the original host plant. By this means, infection intensifies within a local area. Late in summer or early fall, the **telial stage** is produced. These are brown hair-like structures that sometimes occur in such numbers as to give a faintly felt-like appearance to the underside of the leaves (fig. 4-3). These structures then germinate in place under proper climatic conditions, giving rise to the **sporidial stage**, which then infect pines, completing the cycle. Infection of pine requires at least 2 days of saturated atmosphere and maximum temperatures not exceeding 68 °F (20 °C). Moist cool weather in summer and fall favor the disease, whereas warm dry weather is unfavorable.

Field identification—On pines, the first noticeable symptoms are tiny yellow spots on the needles. The spots later turn golden yellow, producing a yellow mottle. As the fungus invades a twig, it too turns yellow. Invasion of branches subsequently occurs from infected twigs. Infection sites then enlarge to produce the spindle-like swellings. Cankers on branches and trunks continue to enlarge from year to year. The invaded bark first becomes yellow or bronzed. The **pycnial stage,** containing an exudate of pycniospores, develops in the swollen tissue. Later aecia are produced in place of the pycnia, and new pycnia appear in the outer margin of infected branch tissue. In spring the aecia appear as raised blisters. They push through the bark to the surface and discharge yellow, dusty masses of aeciospores.

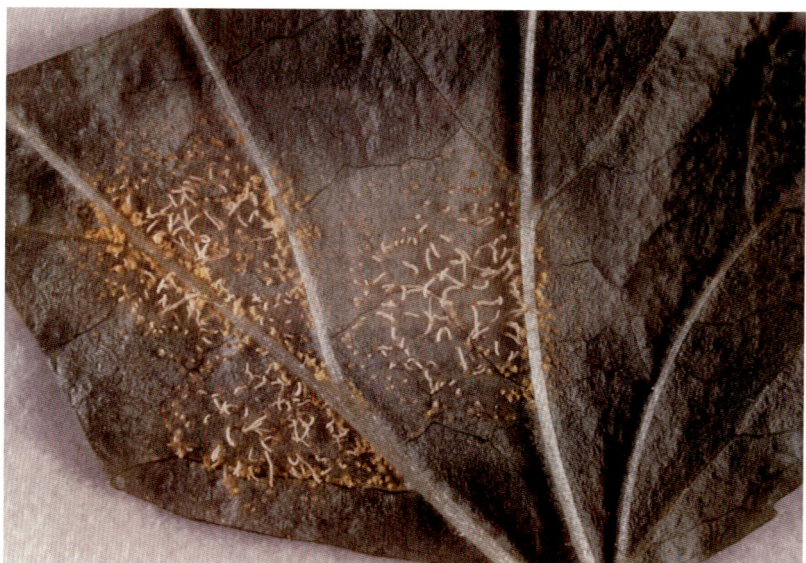

Figure 4-3—Ribes *leaf showing uredinial pustules and telial horns of white pine blister rust.*

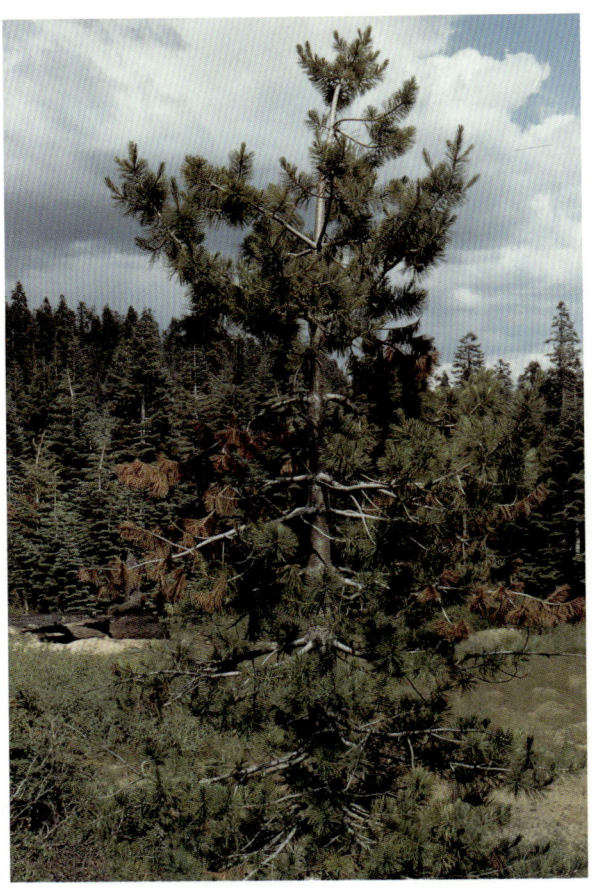

Figure 4-4—*Multiple branch flagging on sugar pine caused by white pine blister rust.*

After the aecia have shed their aeciospores, the bark tissue dies. As a canker progresses, it will have four zones: a yellow zone, a zone showing pycnia, a zone bearing aecia, and an inner area of dead bark where aecia have formed in the previous season. A common symptom in pines first noticeable to the casual observer is branch killing or flagging after the fungus has completely girdled the branch and killed the cambium (fig. 4-4).

On *Ribes*, the uredia appear as slightly raised yellow spots on the lower side of the leaves, petioles, and young stems. Telia, which follow uredia, are darker, and the teliospores are borne in columns up to 2 mm in length. Heavy infection on some *Ribes* hosts such as *R. roezli* may cause premature defoliation. In the western United States, *C. ribicola* is frequently confused with the native rust, *C. occidentale* (see pinyon blister rust). On *Ribes*, the two fungi cannot be separated macroscopically. This similarity has caused a great deal of confusion in attempts to determine the distribution of *C. ribicola* on *Ribes* species in a given year.

Native Limb and Canker Rusts of Pines
Cronartium coleosporioides

Taxonomic knowledge of this group of fungi, sometimes referred to as part of the *Cronartium coleosporioides* complex, is still incomplete. This handbook follows nomenclature based on the imperfect (aecial) stage of the fungus. Effects on pine hosts are classified for field identification as to whether infection results in cankers, galls, or limb rust. This classification, however, does not separate the causal fungi; for example, gall fungi all cause cankers, too. Even though they infect only current-season's growth, they may, depending on host species attacked, become systemic and cause cankers or galls on the main stem of the tree. Until the taxonomy is better understood, two distinct species—*Peridermium stalactiforme* (stalactiform rust) and *P. filamentosum* (filamentosum rust)—are considered to cause limb rust on pine.

Stalactiform Rust
Peridermium stalactiforme

Hosts—The principal pine hosts of *P. stalactiforme* are lodgepole, Jeffrey, and ponderosa pines. In the Laguna Mountains in San Diego County, *P. stalactiforme* has been found on Coulter pine. Its alternate hosts are in the figwort family (Scrophulariaceae), particularly *Castilleja* species (Indian paintbrush).

Distribution and damage—Stalactiform rust occurs from the southwestern United States and California, northward into Canada, and eastward into Michigan, and the Maritime Provinces of Canada.

P. stalactiforme causes cankers on most of its hosts but is known to cause limb rust on Jeffrey pine only from Plumas County southward to San Diego County in California, and in Washoe, Ormsby, and Douglas Counties in Nevada. Whether it also causes limb rust in ponderosa pine is uncertain. *P. stalactiforme* in the Sierra Nevada usually occurs on immature pines in concentrated infection centers and often in close proximity to its alternate host. Most infections are found low in the tree crown.

In the western United States, the main damage is from trunk cankers and resulting cull in lodgepole pine. Stalactiform rust can kill trees by girdling, but this is uncommon except in seedlings or where two or more cankers coalesce. Infected branches are occasionally killed, but no appreciable loss in growth is known.

Disease cycle—In late summer and fall, the airborne sporidia infect susceptible pines. Although rarely seen, pycnia may appear the following spring or one or more years later, depending on the age of

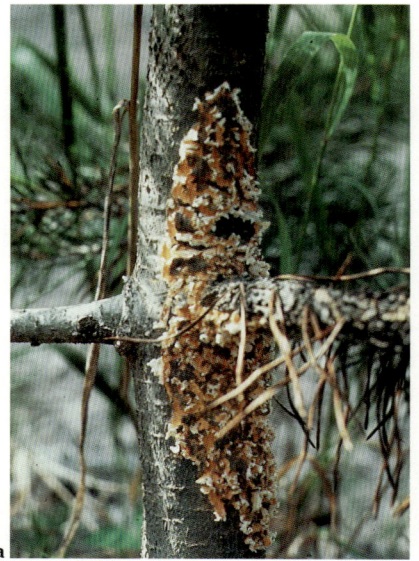 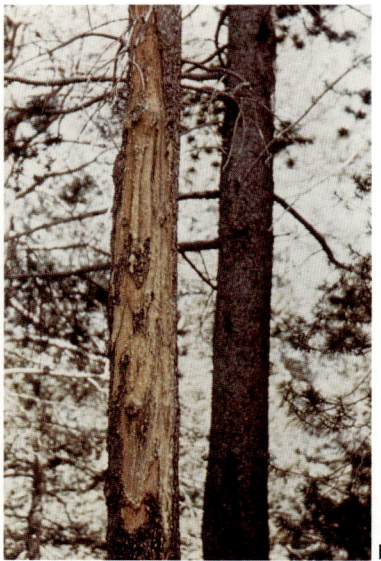

Figure 4-5—*A young sporulating canker of* Peridermium stalactiforme, *on lodgepole pine (**a**). An old, elongate canker of stalactiform rust on lodgepole pine (**b**).*

the pine and its environment. Aecia then appear during the same season but frequently do not mature until early spring of the following year. The aeciospores are not known to infect pine but readily infect the telial host *(Castilleja)* and can be windborne for great distances. Uredia are produced on the telial hosts a few weeks after infection. Urediospores are windborne short distances and serve to intensify the disease on the host or to spread the disease to nearby host plants. They cannot infect pine, however. Telia then appear on the host later in summer and early fall. The teliospores germinate in place and produce sporidia. The sporidia then are windborne short distances to nearby susceptible pines.

Field identification—On most hosts, branch swelling and cankers that finally become much longer than wide are common. On Jeffrey pine, fungus growth becomes systemic, and limb rust results. Multiple swellings are occasionally found on branches with systemic infections. In stem and branch tissues, the fungus spreads much slower laterally than longitudinally (fig. 4-5a). On the trunks of older lodgepole pines, the fungus typically causes elongated or sunken cankers up to 30 feet (9 m) or more long (fig. 4-5b). Each year, cankers grow several inches vertically but only about 0.2 to 0.5 inch (0.05 to 1.3 cm) horizontally. Because rodents usually chew the canker margins, aecia are not easily seen on older trunk cankers. Pines are more frequently infected with stalactiform rust than with comandra rust or filamentosum limb rust. Symptoms and signs on the alternate host are similar to those described for white pine blister rust.

In Jeffrey pines stalactiform rust mainly attacks the lower crowns. The fungus spreads slowly and in some trees does not keep up with stem growth. Thus, when mature infected pines are found, the infection is usually several decades old. Stalactiform rust has been found occasionally in mid-crowns or upper crowns of mature trees in southern California.

Both *P. stalactiforme* and *P. filamentosum* may occur as a limb rust in the same stands of Jeffrey pine in some areas. Stalactiform rust may be distinguished from that caused by *P. filamentosum* by (1) fungus morphology, notably the lower more confluent aecia and the thick smooth areas on aeciospore walls of *P. stalactiforme,* (2) lack of peridial fragments retained on infected twigs from previous year's growth of aecia, (3) the constant presence of rough bark on cankers, and (4) more defined canker development.

Filamentosum Rust
Peridermium filamentosum

Hosts—*Peridermium filamentosum* has the following pine hosts: Apache, Jeffrey, and ponderosa. One form is heteroecious on *Castilleja* species. Two other forms, also called *P. filamentosum,* appear to spread directly from pine to pine without requiring the alternate host.

Distribution and damage—Filamentosum rust is found in California, the southwestern United States, and from western South Dakota and northeastern Utah southward to Colorado, New Mexico, and Arizona. In California, it has been found in the Sierra Nevada from Plumas County to northern Baja California, Mexico. No intense outbreaks of this rust have been found in species other than ponderosa and Jeffrey pines. Because little is known of its epidemiology, its potential importance cannot be fully gauged.

Disease cycle—The life cycle of *P. filamentosum* is almost identical to that of *P. stalactiforme. P. filamentosum,* however, consists of at least three races in the western United States. One race alternates with *Castilleja* species, thereby resembling *P. stalactiforme* in life cycle. Alternate hosts are unknown for the other two races. The second race attacks ponderosa pine in Utah and adjacent states. The third is found on Jeffrey pine. In California, aecia of *P. filamentosum* begin to emerge in the Sierra Nevada during early spring at low elevations but are produced mainly in late June and July. Commonly, aecia may be found still intact in August and retain their spores until September.

Field identification—*P. filamentosum* commonly attacks mid-crowns or upper crowns of mature trees (fig. 4-6a). The aecia on infected branches are noticeably longer and thinner than those of

Figure 4-6—
Filamentosum rust, Peridermium filamentosum, *nearly always infects in the mid-crown or upper crown of trees and spreads in both directions (***a***). The aecia of filamentosum rust on Jeffrey pine are noticeably longer than those produced by stalactiform rust (***b***).*

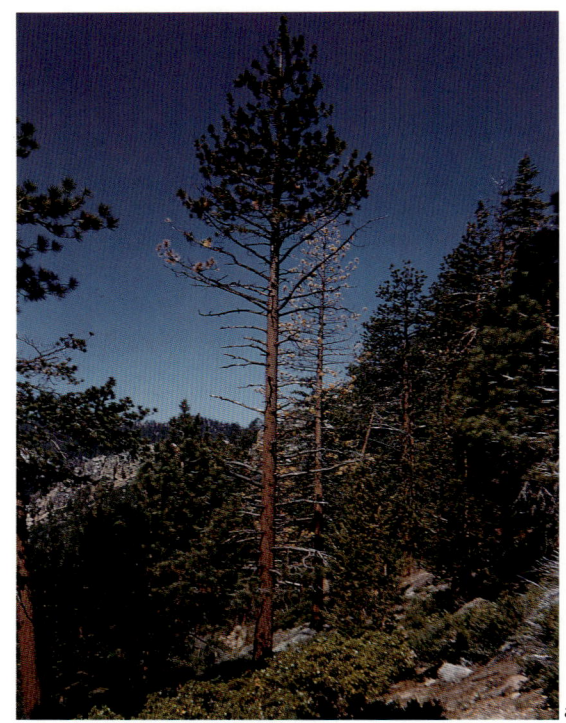

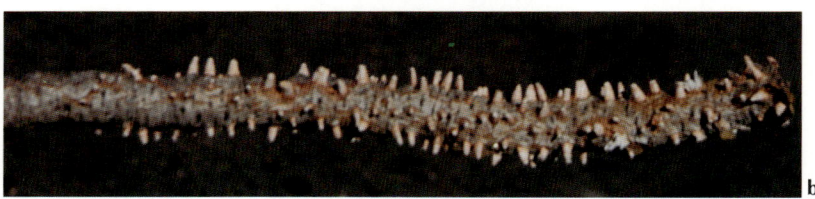

P. stalactiforme (fig. 4-6b). In the Sierra Nevada, the rust is usually found in scattered, mature, and overmature pines, although occasional concentrations occur without apparent reference to stand condition or topography. (See the section on stalactiform rust for help in identifying this species.)

Western Gall Rust
Peridermium harknessii

Hosts—Throughout its range, *P. harknessii* has been found on 22 pine species, which represent 8 of the 9 subsections of hard pines. It is especially common on Monterey, lodgepole, and ponderosa pines.

Distribution and damage—Western gall rust ranges from Mexico to Alaska and eastward in North America to the mid-Atlantic areas.

In the Pacific States, it is widespread and occurs on nearly all of the species of hard pines. It is especially prominent on Monterey pine in both its natural range and wherever it has been planted, and on lodgepole pine along the Pacific Coast, throughout the Sierra Nevada, and on the east side of the Cascade Range in Oregon and Washington.

This rust damages pines by (1) killing seedlings, (2) producing branch galls so numerous that larger trees are killed outright or their growth is diminished by loss of branches, and (3) producing trunk cankers so deforming that they reduce the strength of the tree and increase the likelihood of wind breakage. Western gall rust is the native stem rust found most often in forest disease surveys. All signs suggest that it will become an even more serious problem in the western United States when plantations become more abundant. It is now a serious problem in Christmas tree plantations and nurseries in the western and eastern United States.

Disease cycle—In spring aecia emerge from the living bark of the globose galls and the marginal swellings of the trunk (hip) cankers. Aeciospores can directly infect other pines. These spores are wind-disseminated and may spread the disease for hundreds of miles or kilometers. Moist conditions favor infection of young pine tissue by the germinating spores.

Field identification—The disease is characterized by the formation of globose to pear-shaped galls as large as 12 inches (30 cm) in diameter on branches and stems of pine of all ages (fig. 4-7). Yellow-orange spore pustules are produced in cracks in the galls in spring and early summer. Trunk or "hip" cankers are common (fig. 4-8). Some brooming and proliferation of lateral branches occur as a result of infection. Each new pine infection is followed by formation of well-delimited globose galls. Thereafter, the galls continue to enlarge and produce new spores each spring until they have girdled and killed the branch or stem. However, the fungus may survive in cankers for up to 200 years before girdling is complete.

Comandra Blister Rust
Cronartium comandrae

Hosts—The rust is a heteroecious fungus whose alternate hosts in the western United States are two species of bastard or false toadflax (*Comandra* spp.). Aecial hosts are hard pines—mainly ponderosa, Jeffrey, lodgepole, knobcone, and Scotch pines. Field evidence, however, shows that lodgepole and ponderosa pines are especially susceptible, whereas Jeffrey and knobcone pines are rarely attacked.

Distribution and damage—The fungus is perennial in trunk cankers or branch swellings. Studies on the chronology of disease outbreaks in California indicate that infection was abundant for

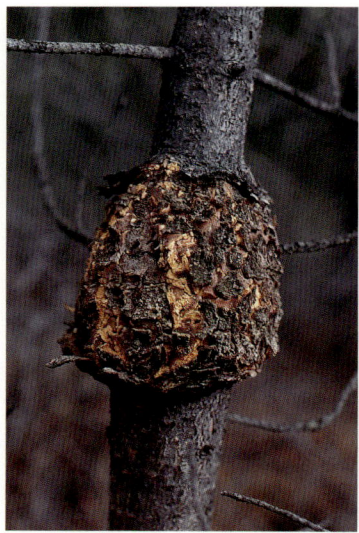 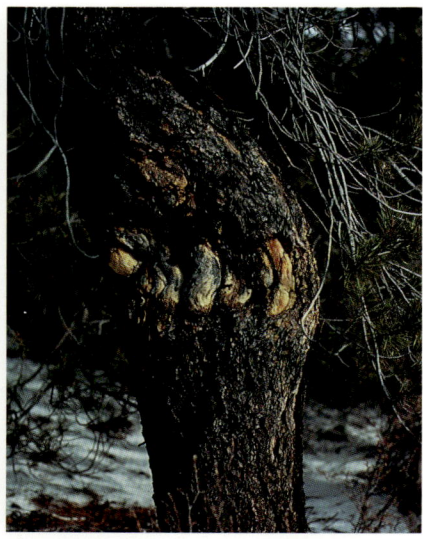

Figure 4-7—*Globose galls of western gall rust are common on lodgepole pine infected by* Peridermium harknessii.

Figure 4-8—*Old but still active hip canker on lodgepole pine caused by western gall rust.*

several years but has become extremely scarce, principally because of extreme fluctuations in the abundance of its alternate host.

The fungus is widely distributed, ranging from Quebec to the Northwest Territory to British Columbia, and southward to New Mexico and California, but has not been found outside of North America. In the western United States, the fungus is found in all States from the Rocky Mountains to the Pacific Ocean. The disease is now common on lodgepole pine in the Rocky Mountains. In California it occurs mainly on ponderosa pine in the Shasta and Klamath River drainages. It is locally common in Oregon and Washington east of the Cascade Range.

Comandra blister rust has been most damaging to lodgepole pine in western Wyoming and the adjacent States, where mortality continues to be heavy as a result of an epidemic that started in the late 1940's. In California the rust is still common in the Shasta River drainage on ponderosa pine even though no outbreak has been recorded since the early 1900's.

Disease cycle—Seasonal activity of the fungus usually starts in late spring with the production of whitish-colored spore sacs (aecia) on the pine cankers. The sacs soon break, releasing many orange-colored spores (aeciospores), which are wind-disseminated to the alternate host, *Comandra*. About 10 days later, the uredial stage forms on the *Comandra* leaves and produces urediospores. These spores can infect other *Comandra* plants. This is the repeating stage of the rust and serves to intensify the disease during the growing season. In early summer the uredial stage is followed by the telial stage. Telial columns grow up to nearly one-tenth inch in length and consist of a mass of teliospores held together in a gelatinous matrix. Teliospores, like those of other *Cronartium*, are dispersed and infect pine hosts.

Moisture and mild temperatures are required for germination of all spore types produced by the fungus and for the subsequent infection of either host. Not every year in which the rust is prevalent on the comandra host is the weather favorable for infection of pines. The lack of recent infection of pines in many parts of the western United States is due, in part, to unfavorable environmental conditions for infection, but when outbreaks occur the disease can be damaging.

Field identification—Comandra rust on hard pines is quite similar to blister rust on white pines in its growth and the damage it causes. The rust causes slight swellings followed by cracking of the infected bark. Small branches or seedling stems are usually girdled quickly as the fungus spreads in the bark and outer wood. Death follows within a few years. The rust eventually encircles trunks or branches, and soon the bark and parts distal to the girdle die. When the fungus reaches large branches or trunks, elongate cankers are formed and copious resin flow from these cankers is common. Rodents usually hasten girdling action by removing bark from cankers. On trunks of older trees with comandra rust, little or no swelling is apparent. Frequently the only symptom is a constriction of the stem with the infected bark becoming roughened. Large ponderosa pines in Oregon often suffer top kill and progressive branch dieback from comandra rust infection (fig. 4-9). Aecia are seldom produced on the trunk cankers in large trees—probably because of the thick bark.

Symptoms on the comandra host are primarily restricted to leaves and occasionally to stems. These appear in the spring as yellowish spots (uredia) about the size of a pin head (fig.4-10). Then, in early summer, brownish hair-like structures or telia develop. Curling and necrosis of heavily infected comandra leaves are common in most areas.

Pinyon Rust
Cronartium occidentale

Hosts—The aecial stage of this rust is found on pinyon and singleleaf pinyons. The telial stage occurs on *Ribes* species.

Distribution and damage—The disease is widespread on *Ribes* along the Pacific Coast but of limited distribution on pines in California. In California infection of pinyons occurs only in a narrow belt, about 50 miles (80 km) long by 10 miles (16 km) wide, stretching south along the border of California and Nevada, on the eastern slope

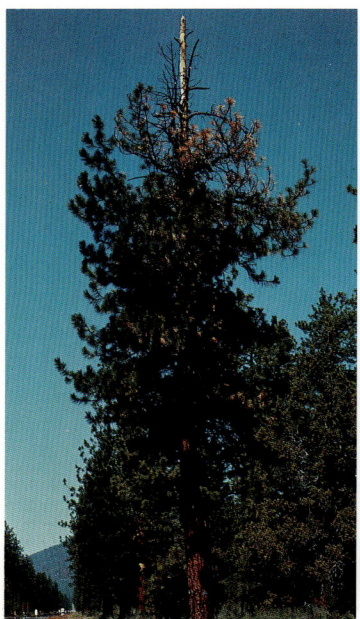

Figure 4-9—*Top kill of ponderosa pine by comandra rust* (Cronartium comandrae).

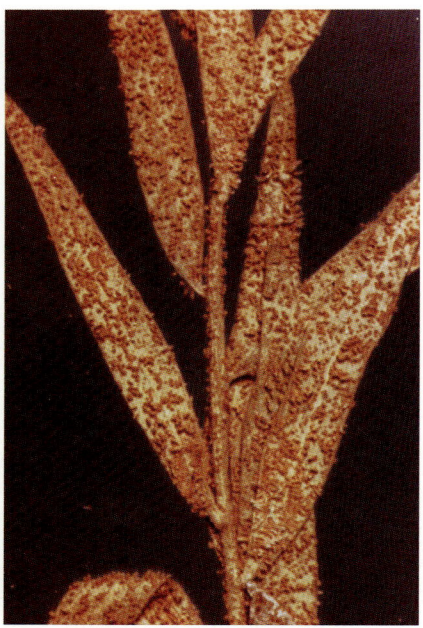

Figure 4-10—*Uredinial and telial stages of comandra rust on bastard toadflax* (Comandra *spp.*).

of the Sierra Nevada from about Gardnerville, Nevada, to north of Bridgeport, CA. From this source of aeciospores, however, annual infection on *Ribes* can be found throughout northern, central, and north coastal California and southern Oregon. On pines, multiple branch and trunk cankers are common and occasionally kill trees. On *Ribes*, damage is restricted to partial defoliation; the plant seldom dies as a result.

Disease cycle—*C. occidentale* is a heteroecious rust fungus with a disease and life cycle identical to that of *C. ribicola*.

Field identification—Because the uredinial and telial stages on *Ribes* are macroscopically indistinguishable from *C. ribicola*, pest control workers in search of *C. occidentale* may have problems in identification.

The aecial stage on the pine host is less distinct than that of *C. ribicola*. It seldom causes swellings on either branches or stems; the orange aeciospores are borne in large irregular cracks in the bark. The aecia themselves are not prominent and seldom visible, in contrast with other stem rusts (see *C. ribicola* and *P. filamentosum*). Rodents often chew on cankers. This characteristic, however, cannot be used as a definite indicator of rust infection.

Sweetfern Rust
Cronartium comptoniae

Host—This rust occurs on lodgepole, Monterey, Jeffrey, and bishop pines in the western United States and on several other pines in other parts of the United States. Its telial hosts are principally sweetfern and sweetgale.

Distribution and damage—The disease is common on 2- and 3-needle pines throughout the eastern United States and Canada, and in the West from Alaska to California. Branch and especially trunk cankers deform trees and frequently kill them. Young trees are more often attacked than older ones. Damage can be extensive in nurseries.

Disease cycle—*C. comptoniae* is a heteroecious rust fungus and, except for differences in aecial and telial hosts, has a life cycle nearly identical to that of *C. ribicola*.

Field identification—The rust on pines usually first becomes evident as elongated swelling on branches of older trees or on the stem of seedlings. These swellings become evident within 1 to 2 years after infection. They are most conspicuous in spring when the orange-yellow aeciospores are formed. Older cankers may vary from deep, vertical fissures to very slight depressions in the bark. The uredial stage appears as orange pustules on the underside of the leaves of sweetfern and sweetgale. In autumn, telia form around and within the uredia.

Tarweed Rust
Coleosporium madiae

Hosts—This heteroecious rust fungus has its aecial stage primarily on Monterey pine, Coulter pine, and Jeffrey pine. The telial hosts are principally *Madia* spp. (tarweed).

Distribution and damage—The rust is found occasionally on its tarweed hosts from British Columbia south to central California. It has not been found on its aecial hosts north of southern Oregon. The fungus is restricted to needles of its conifer hosts and, except in occasional wet years when it may build up and cause heavy defoliation, damage is minimal. On its telial hosts, damage is also minimal.

Field identification—Aecia occur on all surfaces of the needle. They are white, globoid, and broadly ellipsoid, and usually appear in early spring (fig. 4-11). On tarweed leaves, uredinia appear as small, round, golden yellow pustules. Telia are waxy, compact, and orange yellow when fresh.

Aster Rust
Coleosporium asterum (C. solidaginis)

Aster rust is one of the most common rusts in the United States. The uredinial stage occurs on species of aster and goldenrod.

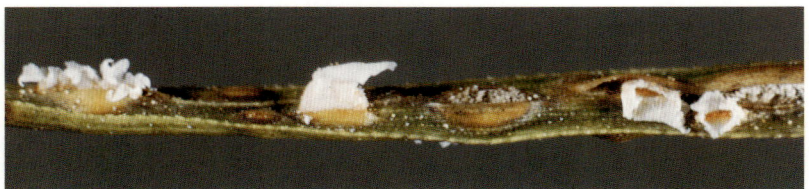

Figure 4-11—*Aecia of tarweed rust* (Coleosporium madiae) *protrude from an infected needle of Monterey pine.*

C. asterum usually overwinters on the rosettes of these species. On its aecial host in the West, it is found mostly on needles of lodgepole pine but occurs only sporadically (fig. 4-12). Damage to the pine host is usually negligible. Symptoms on pine are discolored spots on needles, with firm, protruding, light-orange aecial sacs (fig. 4-13). On aster and goldenrod, the uredinia are round, orange-yellow pustules on the leaves, whereas the telia are scattered and reddish orange, with cylindrical teliospores rounded at both ends.

RUSTS ON FIR AND DOUGLAS-FIR

Several needle rusts infect true firs in western North America. Except for *Melampsorella caryophyllacearum*, however, most of them are usually of minor importance and scattered in incidence except in Christmas tree plantations. The two most common are *Pucciniastrum goeppertianum* and *Pucciniastrum epilobii*. On Douglas-fir and bigcone Douglas-fir, only two rusts of any significance in western United States have been reported: *Melampsora medusae* and *Melampsora occidentalis*. Both alternate between needles of Douglas-fir and leaves of poplars and aspens.

Yellow Witches-Broom of Fir
Melampsorella caryophyllacearum

Hosts—*Melampsorella caryophyllacearum*, the fungus causing yellow witches-broom, has as its aecial host the true firs. In western United States, these tree species are principally white fir, California red fir, grand fir, and subalpine fir. Trees of all ages are susceptible to the parasite. The alternate hosts are several species of *Stellaria* (chickweed) and *Cerastium* (mouse-ear chickweed).

Distribution and damage—*M. caryophyllacearum* is found on fir species in North America from Labrador and Newfoundland west to Alaska, south through Canada to the northern United States and in the western United States, and from California to Mexico. The disease is abundant in southern Idaho, western Wyoming, and northern Utah on subalpine fir, and in the south and central Sierra Nevada of California on red fir. Elsewhere in the western United States, brooms are only

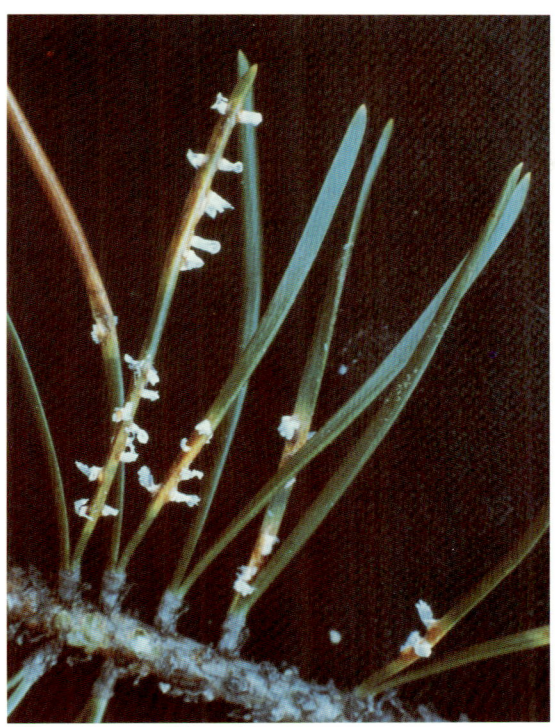

Figure 4-12—*In aster rust, the empty aecia of Coleosporium asterum, are still evident on the infected needles of lodgepole pine.*

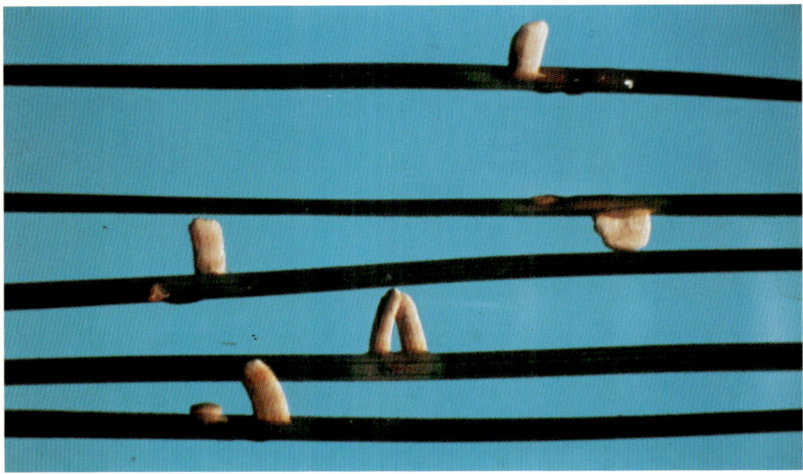

Figure 4-13—*Mature aecia of the aster rust protrude from an infected needle of lodgepole pine.*

occasionally found. Most of the infected trees have branch brooms and, less frequently, trunk burls or spike tops. Multiple brooms can reduce tree growth, provide infection courts for heartrots, and even kill trees—particularly seedlings and saplings.

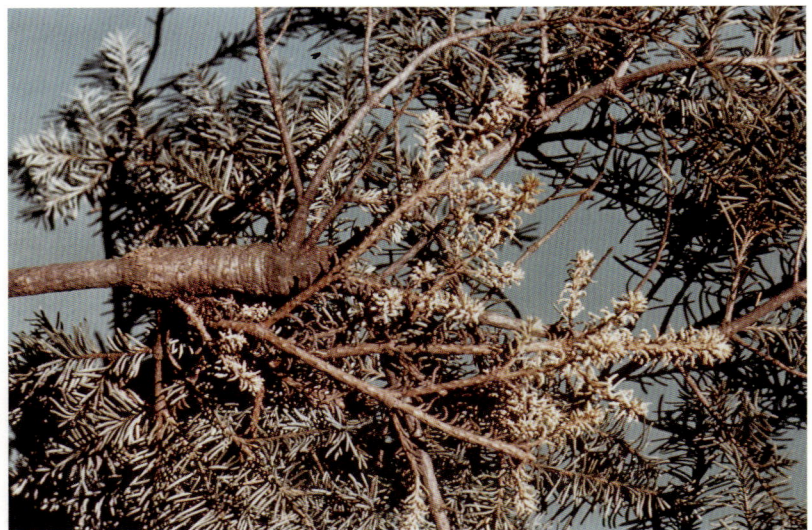

Figure 4-14—*Witches-broom of white fir caused by fir broom rust (*Melampsorella caryophyllacearum*) showing compact growth and light-colored, infected needles.*

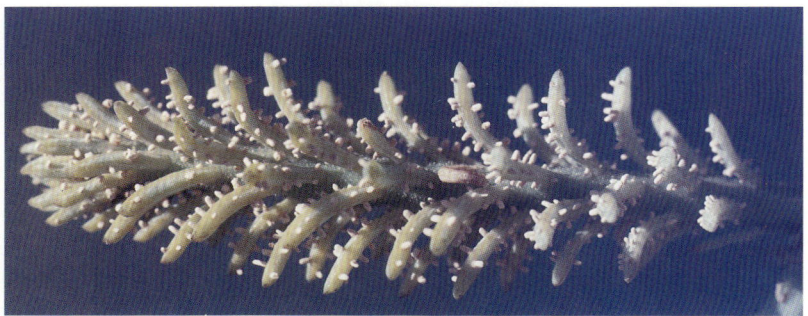

Figure 4-15—*Light-colored aecial pustules of the fir broom rust on infected needles of California red fir.*

Disease cycle—*M. caryophyllacearum* is a heteroecious rust, alternating between true firs and chickweeds. The fungus is systemic and perennial, not only on its aecial host (true firs) but also on its telial host. True firs are probably infected in the spring, when airborne basidiospores land on and penetrate newly emerging twig and bud tissue. The alternate hosts are infected in summer or fall, when aeciospores released from infected firs land on developing foliage. Moist conditions favor infection on both hosts.

Field identification—The most noticeable characteristic of this disease is the witches-broom it produces. The brooms are most conspicuous from mid-summer to late fall, when their yellowish-

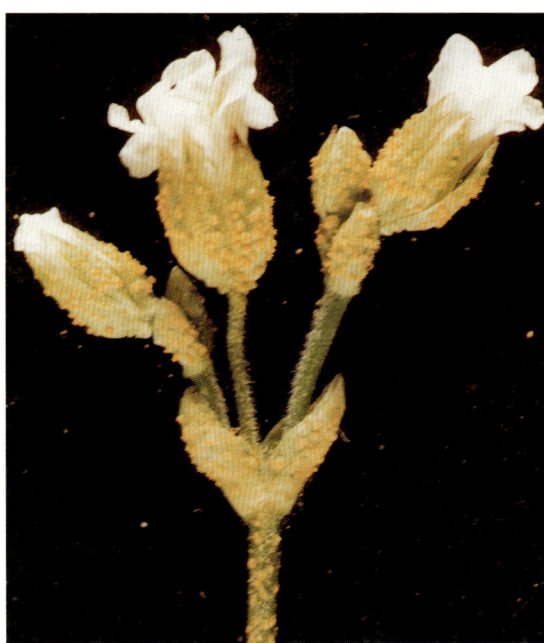

Figure 4-16—*Yellow uredia cover the floral structure of a chickweed infected by fir broom rust.*

orange color reaches a peak of intensity and stands out in striking contrast to the normal dark green foliage (fig. 4-14). Aecia on the diseased needles contribute to this color. Witches-brooms are upright, typically compact, and have a dense growth of many small and shortened branches that rarely exceed 3 feet (1 m) in diameter. The diseased needles are greatly shortened and thickened (fig. 4-15). In winter the brooms appear to be dead—the affected needles shrivel and become dark. In autumn the needles drop, leaving the brooms bare until new growth starts. The new needles are yellowish green until mid-summer. On the alternate host—chickweed—the fungus forms the uredial and telial stages (fig. 4-16). The abundance of fir broom rust appears to be related to change in abundance of the alternate host. Specific conditions for infection are responsible for very sporadic outbreaks of disease on true firs.

Fir Blueberry Rust
Pucciniastrum goeppertianum

The hosts are true firs and blueberry. On true fir, *P. goeppertianum* forms white tubules on the lower side of needles (fig. 4-17). These tubules contain orange powdery aeciospores. Frequently witches-brooms with annual needles form on true firs. Uredia are absent on blueberry species. On blueberry, the telia form

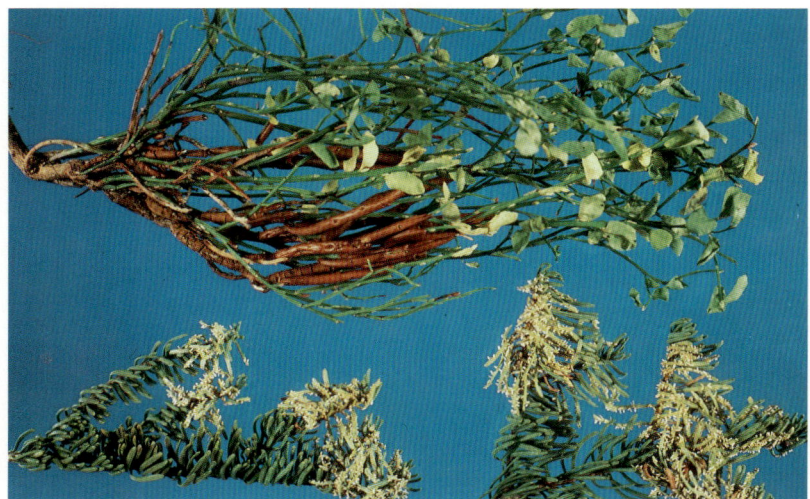

Figure 4-17—*In fir-blueberry rust,* Puccniastrum goeppertianum *infects both blueberry and true firs. The swollen, reddish stems of blueberry are infected by the telial stage of the fungus, whereas the aecial stage indicated by the elongate, yellowish aecia infects needles of true firs.*

a continuous layer around the stem and appear as a polished reddish-brown surface (fig. 4-17). Witches-broom development on blueberry is common. Teliospores are found within the epidermis in single, closely pressed layers.

Fir Willow Weed Rust
(Pucciniastrum epilobii)

This disease is scattered but not uncommon on true fir species throughout the western United States. The fungus is also known as *Pucciniastrum pustulatum.* The aecia are elongate, cylindric, yellow to colorless pustules on the leaves of fir (fig. 4-18). On the alternate host, *Salix* spp. (willows), uredia appear as powdery orange-yellow pustules on the developing leaves. Telia, which are reddish-brown to blackish-brown crusts, overwinter in the dead leaves.

Douglas-fir Rust
(Melampsora medusae) (M. albertensis)

Distributed throughout western United States from Colorado and Wyoming to British Columbia and Oregon, and into California, Douglas-fir rust has also been found on bigcone Douglas-fir in southern California. The fungus is also known as *M. albertensis.* On Douglas-fir, the aecia form as 1 mm long tubules in two rows—one

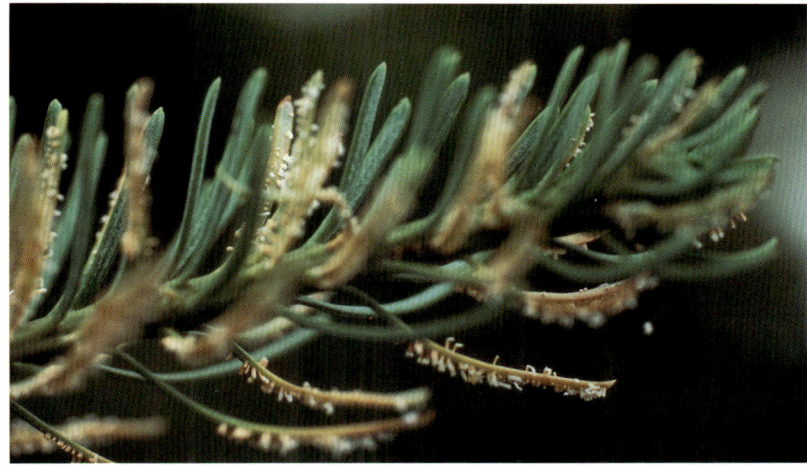

Figure 4-18—*Light-colored, cylindrical aecia are produced on needles of true firs infected by willow weed rust* (Pucciniastrum epilobii).

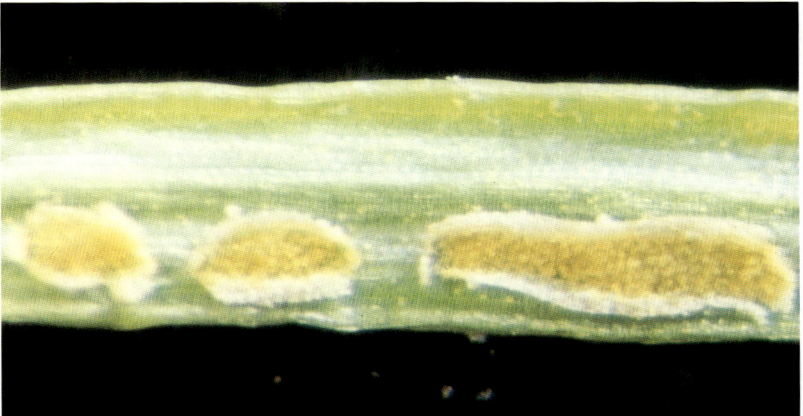

Figure 4-19—*Aecia of Douglas-fir rust* (Melampsora medusae) *appear as elongate pustules on either side of infected Douglas-fir needles.*

on either side of the mid-rib of the needle (fig. 4-19). These tubules contain powdery yellow spores which, in turn, infect leaves of the alternate host, *Populus* species (cottonwood and poplar). The uredial stage of the rust on cottonwood and poplar appears as powdery yellow pustules on the lower leaf surface. Later, these pustules become waxy, orange-brown mats under the epidermis, forming the telial stage.

RUSTS ON INCENSE-CEDAR AND JUNIPERS

A large number of rusts, primarily in the genus *Gymnosporangium,* are found scattered throughout the western United States and, although they cause little damage to forest stands, they can cause considerable damage to ornamental plantings.

Incense-Cedar Rust
Gymnosporangium libocedri

Hosts—One of the most abundant rust fungi on conifers in the western United States, *G. libocedri,* alternates between incense-cedar and rosaceous shrubs, predominantly *Amalanchier* spp. (serviceberry). It causes only minor damage except on the leaves and fruits of serviceberry and hawthorn. This rust is occasionally found on apple, pear, quince, and mountain ash.

Distribution and damage—The disease caused by *G. libocedri* is found throughout the range of incense-cedar in the western United States. It infects incense-cedar of all ages. The fungus seldom kills branches, except for small ones. Often the mycelium penetrates an older twig, resulting in a typical witches-broom. Heavily infected trees bear many brooms and may be seriously weakened, but few trees die of this disease. An infection in the main stem of incense-cedar may result in burls that cause defect in lumber. The rust has caused some damage to commercial pear orchards in northern California and has also been reported on pears in Oregon.

Disease cycle and field identification—*G. libocedri* is a heteroecious rust fungus alternating between incense-cedar and several members of the rose family. In contrast to the other major heteroecious rusts described in this chapter, *G.libocedri* has its pycnial and aecial stages on rosaceous hosts; it lacks a uredial stage and the telial stage is on the conifer host. In early spring small infected branches of incense-cedar trees appear slightly discolored. On the underside (rarely on the upperside) of the green, flat, scale-like leaves, a number of small brown to brick-colored tufts or telial cushions appear (fig. 4-20). When they mature, the cushions become gelatinous during wet periods in spring and finally form conspicuous light orange masses (fig. 4-21) that later dry to a thin film. The sporidial stage is blown to the rosaceous host, where small, orange, cup-shaped fruiting bodies appear on the leaves, petioles, and sometimes the fruit. These fruiting bodies produce the aeciospores, which infect incense-cedar. Moist conditions favor infection.

Witches-brooms caused by *G. libocedri* are frequently mistaken for plants of the incense-cedar mistletoe (fig. 4-22). This mistletoe, however, always hangs down in thick clusters, whereas the bushy witches-brooms caused by the rusts are more or less erect.

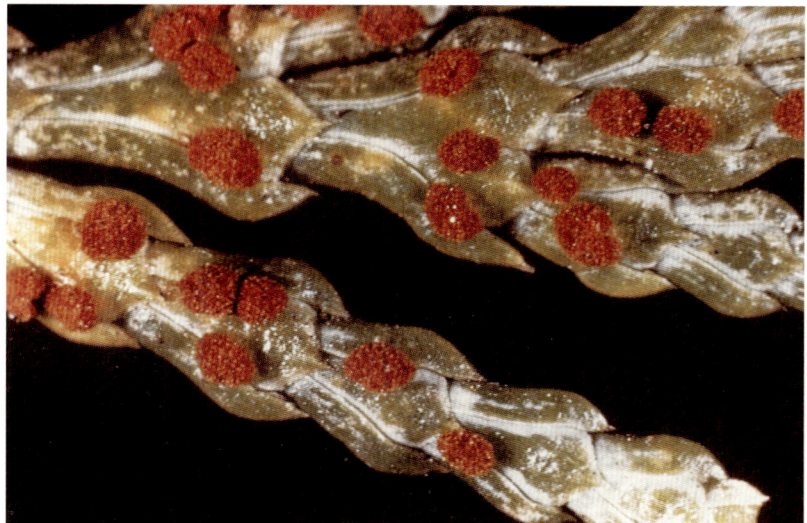

Figure 4-20—*Telial cushions of incense-cedar rust (Gymnosporangium libocedri) on scale-like leaves of incense-cedar.*

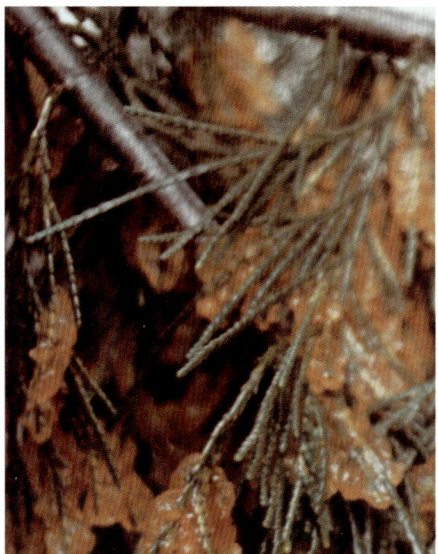

Figure 4-21—*Gelatinous telial stage of incense-cedar rust on incense-cedar.*

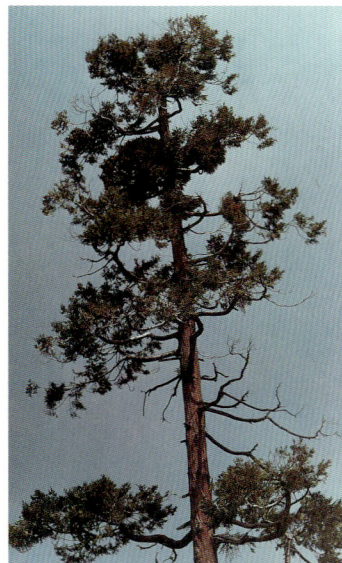

Figure 4-22—*The tight, dark green brooms on incense-cedar are caused by incense-cedar rust. The globose pendant plants on branches are incense-cedar mistletoe.*

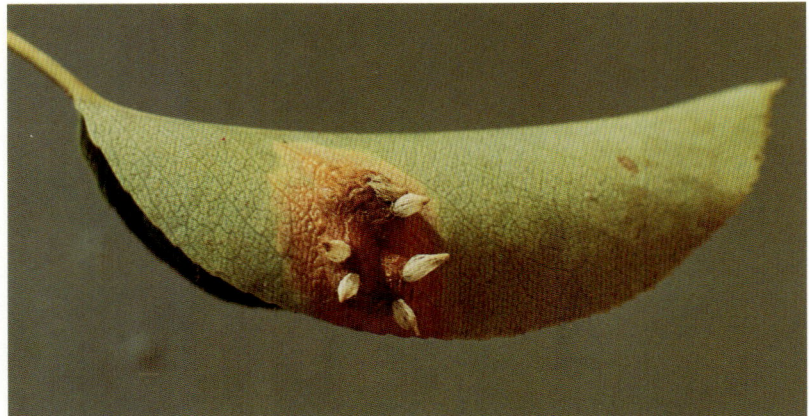

Figure 4-23—*The aecia of* Gymnosporangium fuscum *appear as white tubules on the swollen, orange surface of an infected pear leaf.*

Pear-Juniper Rust
Gymnosporangium fuscum

This disease was found for the first time in California in 1960 on several ornamental juniper plantings and on pear trees in one area. Although damage can be severe on juniper hosts, the greatest economic damage occurs on the pear host. The growth and fruit set of heavily infected trees are reduced, and infected leaves tend to fall early in the season. The fungus also attacks the fruit. On junipers, the telial stage appears on branches and twigs, causing very slight to fusiform swellings several inches long. The perennial infection in junipers often kills the infected branch or twig in 3 to 4 years. The telia occur in horns, small, firm, dark-brown bodies a few millimeters across. Under moist conditions, the horns appear reddish-brown, swell, and become gelatinous. On pears the aecial stage first appears as circular or irregularly shaped yellow-orange spots up to 2 cm in diameter on the lower surface of the leaves. The mature aecial stage appears as orange-brown cushions of diseased tissue, with the aecium an off-white, acorn-shaped tubule 2 to 5 mm high (fig. 4-23).

Amelanchier Rust
Gymnosporangium harknessianum

This rust is found chiefly on western juniper in California and central Oregon. Its alternate host is primarily western serviceberry. On juniper hosts, uredia have not been found. Telia form as reddish-brown gelatinous masses on juniper leaves. Aecia are found chiefly on western serviceberry fruits, usually over the entire surface. They are cinnamon-brown, cylindrical tubules, 4 to 7 mm tall.

Inconspicuous Juniper Rust
Gymnosporangium inconspicuum

Probably the most abundant *Gymnosporangium* on juniper and on serviceberry in the western United States, this rust is found primarily on Utah juniper and western juniper.

On the juniper host, uredia have not been found. Telia are golden yellow to brown felt-like structures arising between the scale-like leaves on green twigs or frequently through the bark of woody twigs. In some parts of Utah and Nevada, the telial stage is common on older branches and larger stems. The host tissue swells slightly, but its bark appears to be abnormally rough. Although telia frequently fall off green twigs after maturation and leave no obvious signs, on woody bark they are often retained in the cracks so that the disease can be diagnosed at any time of the year. The fungus can also cause woody swellings, but these are rare. The aecial stage on the serviceberry host is chiefly on the fruits. Aecia appear as pale yellow, oblong cylindrical tubules. In some areas, fruits may be so heavily infected that almost none mature. Infected fruits are often colored bright yellow or orange by the rust, so that the whole bush may appear at first glance to bear yellow or orange fruit.

Serviceberry Rust
Gymnosporangium kernianum

Serviceberry rust is common on several species of juniper throughout the western United States. Its principal conifer hosts are Utah, California, and western junipers. Its principal alternate hosts are serviceberry species, but it is also found on pears, hawthorns, and quinces. On conifer hosts, uredia are not found. Telia are found developing between the scale-like juniper leaves as globose witches-brooms caused by fungus infection. Telia are hemispheric, and dark reddish-brown. On the alternate host, aecia are found principally on leaves and occasionally on fruits and leaf petioles. The aecia are usually inconspicuous, cylindrical, cinnamon-brown pustules. They are sometimes found in mixed infections among the larger, brighter, more abundant aecia of *G. inconspicuum* on the same fruits of serviceberry.

Juniper Rust
Gymnosporangium multiporum

This rust is a seldom-collected species and is of unknown life cycle. It occurs on western juniper in California and on oneseed and Utah junipers in Colorado, New Mexico, and central California. An alternate host for the pycnial and aecial stages is not known. On the juniper host, uredia have not been found. Telia develop between the scale-like leaves on green branches. They are chestnut brown with oblong teliospores.

Nelson's Juniper Rust
Gymnosporangium nelsonii

This rust is found frequently throughout the western United States on creeping, oneseed, western, Rocky Mountain, California, and Utah junipers. Uredia are not found on the conifer host. The telia, however, cause conspicuous woody, globose galls of varying size on branches and small stems. The telia are chestnut brown, irregularly flattened, 3 to 5 mm high. The alternate hosts are principally species of serviceberry, on which the aecia are found on leaves, petioles, and fruits. They are cylindrical, 2 to 4 mm high, with chestnut-brown pustules.

Hawthorn-Juniper Rust
Gymnosporangium confusum

This fungus is found only in one area of California but is common in Eurasia on several telial and aecial hosts. In a restricted area of California, it has become well established on Utah juniper, its telial host, and on oneseed hawthorn, which is the aecial host. Telia develop first as gelatinous horns in spring. When dry, the horns become very dark, velvety, reddish-brown. The horns develop principally in fusiform cortical swellings on woody branches. Pycnia and later aecia develop on swellings of the leaves, petioles, succulent stems, pedicels, and calyxes. Aeciospores are reddish brown and begin to develop usually in May.

RUSTS ON CYPRESS

Two distinct species of rust fungi are found on cypress in the western United States: *Gymnosporangium cupressi* and *Uredio cupressicola*. Both occur only rarely.

Gymnosporangium cupressi

This fungus has been reported on Arizona and Baker cypress in the telial stages and on serviceberry species in the aecial stage. The telial stage causes elongate or globoid swellings on cypress, often in rows on larger branches and forms irregularly wedge-shaped, chestnut-brown telial pustules. Although most common on green twigs, all stages of gall and canker development to ages 100 years or more have been found. The old cankers resemble the hip cankers of *Peridermium harknessii* on pine, with flaring sides of mostly uninfected tissue.

Uredio cupressicola

Only the uredial stage of this fungus has been found, and only on Gowan cypress and Arizona cypress variety *montana*. The rust has been found only in California and Baja California. The uredinia first appear between the scale leaves of young twigs without producing any perceptible swelling. Later large fusiform swellings are evident on twigs 4 years old or older. Cankers usually kill the twigs within a few years but occasionally occur on branches up to 25 years old.

RUSTS ON SPRUCE

Inland Spruce Cone Rust
Chrysomyxa pirolata
Coastal Spruce Cone Rust
Chrysomyxa monesis

Hosts—The primary hosts of these two spruce cone rusts are spruces; alternate hosts are wintergreen *(Pyrola* sp.*)* and single delight *(Monesis uniflora).*

Distribution and damage—Spruce cone rusts occur sporadically in spruce stands in the Pacific Northwest. They can cause considerable damage to spruce seed crops in local areas.

Disease cycle—Both spruce and one of the alternate hosts are required for completion of the life cycle of the pathogen. Perennial infections and continuing urediospore production favor long-term survival and inoculum buildup on the alternate hosts. Spores that infect both primary and alternate hosts are windborne, and moist conditions in summer favor spore germination and subsequent infection.

Field Identification—On spruce, *C. pirolata* or *C. monesis* cause browning of cones, premature cone opening, and destruction of the seed. Yellow aecial spore masses develop between cone scales. On wintergreen and single delight, the pathogens may cause no visible symptoms or there may be slight atrophy and chlorosis. Yellow spore pustules (both uredia and telia) may be observed on any parts of the plants in spring, summer, and fall.

Spruce Broom Rust
Chrysomyxa arctostaphyli

Hosts—The aecial hosts of this rust are spruces; the telial host is bearberry (kinnikinnick) *(Arctostaphylos uva-ursi).*

Distribution and damage—Spruce broom rust is occasionally found in spruce stands in the Pacific Northwest but is seldom damaging. The rust is more common on interior Engelmann spruce. Broom rust has sometimes been mistaken for dwarf mistletoe, but spruces are not commonly infected by dwarf mistletoe.

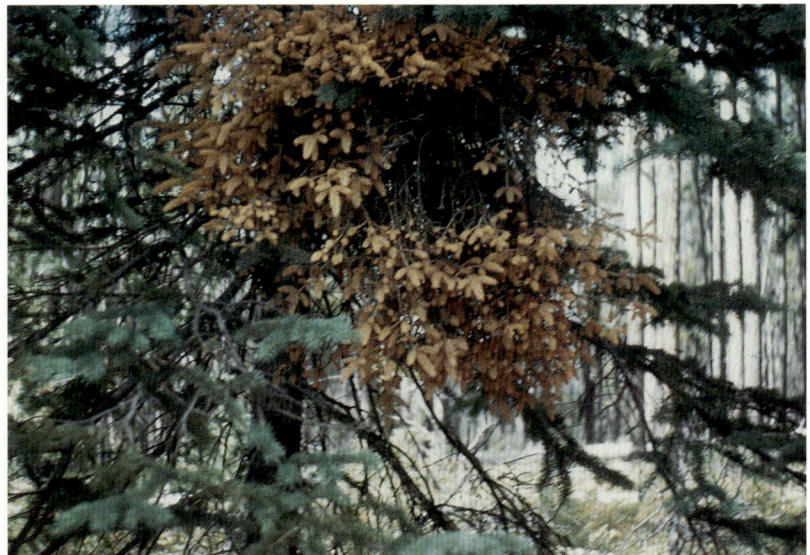

Figure 4-24—*A large broom on Engelmann spruce caused by spruce broom rust* (Chrysomyxa arctostaphyli).

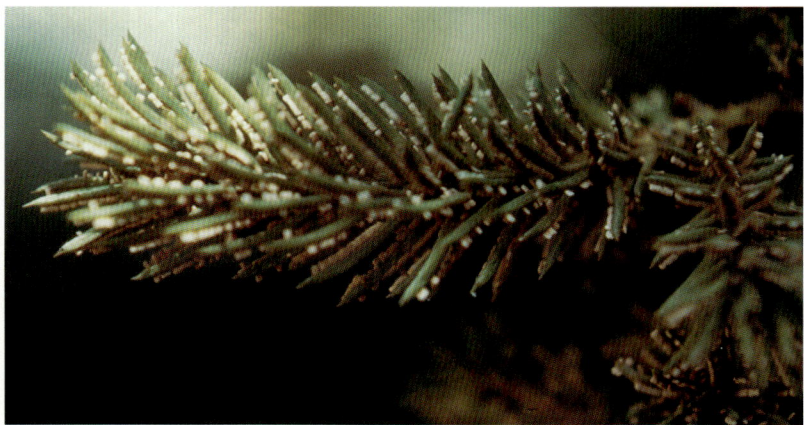

Figure 4-25—*Aecia of spruce broom rust appear as yellow pustules on the surface of infected Engelmann spruce needles.*

Disease cycle—Both spruce and bearberry hosts are required for completion of the life cycle. Spores that infect both hosts are windborne, and moist conditions greatly favor infection.

Field identification—On spruce, *C. arctostaphyli* causes conspicuous witches-brooms with abundant production of short twigs (fig. 4-24). Foliage on witches-brooms is chlorotic and in summer is covered with whitish-yellow aecial pustules (fig. 4-25). These needles die and are shed in the fall, leaving the witches-brooms to appear dead through the winter. On bearberry, *C. arctostaphyli* causes a purple-brown leaf spot. Orange telial pustules develop on the underside of bearberry leaves in late spring.

SELECTED REFERENCES

Arthur, J.C. 1934, 1962. Manual of the rusts of the United States and Canada. 2d ed. New York: Hafner Publishing Co. for Lafayette-Purdue Research Foundation. 438 p.

Bega, R.V. 1959. The capacity and period of maximum production of sporidia in *Cronartium ribicola*. Phytopathology 49(1):51–57.

Bega, R.V. 1960. The effect of environment on germination of sporidia in *Cronartium ribicola*. Phytopathology 50(1):61–69.

Kimmey, James W.; Wagener, Willis W. 1961. Spread of white pine blister rust from ribes to sugar pine in California and Oregon. Tech. Bull. 1251. Washington, DC: U.S. Department of Agriculture. 71 p.

Krebill, R.G. 1965. Comandra rust outbreaks in lodgepole pine. Journal of Forestry 63:519–522.

Krebill, R.G. 1968. *Cronartiam comandrae* in the Rocky Mountain States. Res. Paper INT-50. Ogden, UT: U.S. Department of Agriculture, Forest Service, Intermountain Forest and Range Experiment Station. 28 p.

McCain, A.H. Rosenburg, D.Y. 1961. Pear-juniper rust, a disease new to California and the United States. California Department of Agriculture Bulletin 50:13–19.

Mielke, J.L. 1913. White pine blister rust in western North America. Yale University School Forestry Bulletin 52:155.

Mielke, J.L. 1952. The rust fungus *Cronartium filamentosum* in Rocky Mountain ponderosa pine. Journal of Forestry 50:365–373.

Mielke, J.L. 1956. The rust fungus *Cronartium filamentosum* in lodgepole pine. Journal of Forestry. 54:518–521.

Mielke, J.L. ; Krebill, R.G.; Powers, H.R. 1968. Comandra blister rust of hard pines. Forest Pest Leafl. 62. Washington, DC: U.S. Department of Agriculture. 4 p.

Peterson, R.S. 1963. Effects of broom rust on spruce and fir. Res. Paper INT–8. Ogden, UT: U.S. Department of Agriculture, Forest Service, Intermountain Forest and Range Experiment Station. 10 p.

Peterson, R.S. 1963. Notes on western rust fungi III. Cronartium. Mycologia 54: 678–684.

Peterson, R.S. 1963. Notes on western rust fungi IV. Mycologia 57:465–471.

Peterson, R.S. 1966. Limb rust damage to pine. Res. Paper INT–31. Ogden, UT: U.S. Department of Agriculture, Forest Service, Intermountain Forest and Range Experiment Station. 10 p.

Peterson, R.S. 1967a. The Peridermium species on pine. Bulletin of the Torrey Botanical Club 94:511–542.

Peterson, Roger S. 1967b. Studies of Juniper rusts in the West. Madrono 19:79–91.

Peterson, R.S. 1967c. Cypress rusts in California and Baja California. Madrono 19:47–54.

Peterson, Roger S. 1968. Limb rust of pine: the causal fungi. Phytopathology 58:309–315.

Peterson, Roger S.; Jewell, F.F. 1968. Status of American stem rusts of pine. Annual Review of Phytopathology 6:23–40.

Ziller, Wolf G. 1974. The tree rusts of Western Canada. Publ. 1329. Victoria, BC: Canadian Forest Service. 272 p.

CHAPTER 5   Mistletoes

Robert F. Scharpf and Frank G. Hawksworth

Research Scientist, Emeritus, formerly Project Leader, Disease Research and Principal Plant Pathologist, Pacific Southwest Research Station, Forest Service, U.S. Department of Agriculture, Albany, CA.
Plant Pathologist, retired, Rocky Mountain Forest and Range Experiment Station, Forest Service, U.S. Department of Agriculture, Fort Collins, CO.

INTRODUCTION

The parasitic flowering plants commonly known as mistletoes are found throughout North America. Two genera of mistletoes grow in the western United States: *Phoradendron* (true mistletoes) and *Arceuthobium* (dwarf mistletoes). The true mistletoes grow on both conifers and broadleaf trees; the dwarf mistletoes grow only on conifers. Male and female flowers are produced on separate plants in both genera.

True mistletoes are large woody plants with mature shoots more than 2 feet (0.6 m) long and 2 inches (5 cm) or more in diameter. Foliage is leafy or scaly. The fruit are white or pink berries. On the Pacific Coast the four true mistletoes on conifers are easily distinguished on the basis of foliage characteristics and the host species.

In contrast, dwarf mistletoes are small plants, with mature shoots less than 6 to 8 inches (15 to 20 cm) long and 2 to 5 mm in diameter. The shoots are non-woody, segmented, and have scalelike leaves. Seeds produced in oval-shaped bicolor fruit are forcibly released when ripe.

Although both mistletoes are damaging parasites of trees, by far the greatest timber loss in coniferous forests of the western United States is attributed to the dwarf mistletoes. Billions of board feet of lumber are lost each year as a result of growth reduction and mortality from these parasites. They also cause serious damage to high-value, high-use forest recreational areas.

TRUE MISTLETOES

The true mistletoes are probably more often seen and recognized than the dwarf mistletoes. Even the leafless true mistletoes usually appear as conspicuous clumps or balls of foliage growing on conifers (fig. 5-1, 5-2). True mistletoes are dependent on their hosts for water and nutrients, but they do photosynthesize. Thus, much of their growth is attributed to their ability to make foodstuffs from water and certain mineral elements provided by the host. In the absence of the aerial portions of the plant, however, the roots remain alive and

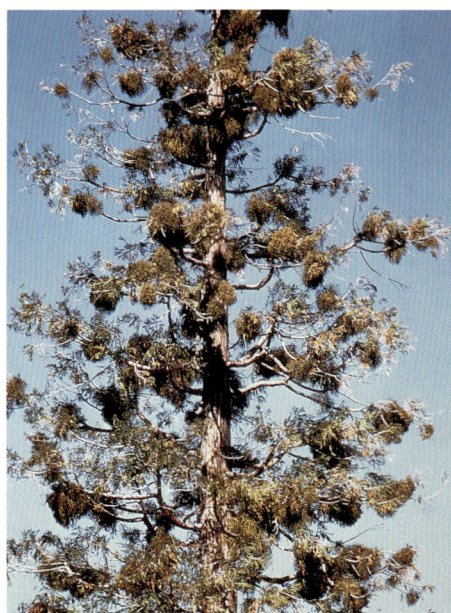

Figure 5-1—*Incense-cedar often becomes severely infected throughout its crown by the incense-cedar mistletoe (*Phoradendron libocedri*).*

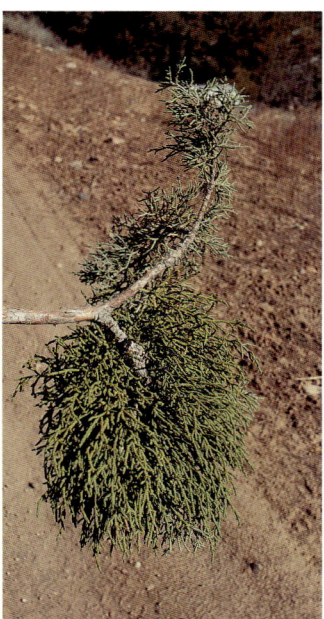

Figure 5-2—*The leafless juniper mistletoe (*Phoradendron juniperinum*) often grows on branches of western juniper.*

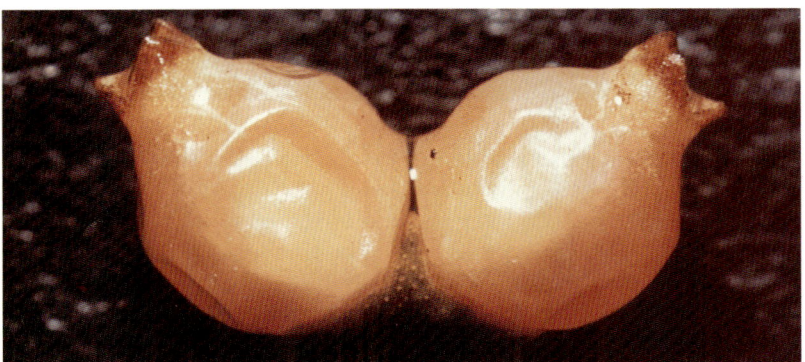

Figure 5-3—*The incense-cedar mistletoe produces round, pinkish fruit about the size of a pea.*

continue to grow within the host branch, eventually producing new shoots and foliage.

Mistletoe flowers are inconspicuous, but the fruits, commonly known as berries, are readily seen (fig. 5-3). They are about the size of a pea (3 to 8 mm) in diameter; when ripe they grow in clusters. Usually one seed develops in each berry. The sticky pulp of the berry

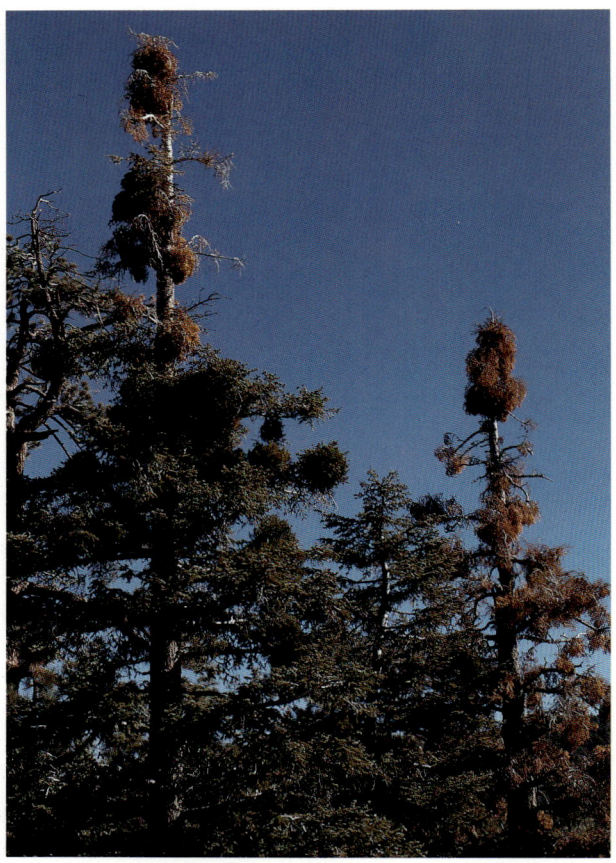

Figure 5-4—
Large clusters of white fir mistletoe (Phoradendron pauciflorum) occur mainly in the tops of mature white fir.

surrounding the seed is a preferred food of several species of birds. When eaten, the seeds pass intact through the digestive tract of the birds and are deposited along with their excrement on tree branches. Consequently, these mistletoes tend to be most abundant in the tops of trees (fig. 5-4). Thread-like strands on the seed coat enable the seeds to adhere to branches, where they germinate, penetrate, and infect the host.

Both the root and shoot systems are initially produced from the germinating seed. Thereafter, buds produced from the roots break through the bark to form additional aerial shoots. Woody perennial stems develop and often persist for many years unless they are broken off or killed. Often clumps of shoots and foliage 2 to 3 feet (0.6 to 0.9 m) in diameter are seen in trees.

The four true mistletoes on conifers on the Pacific Coast are easy to identify. They may be distinguished on the basis of foliage and host species with the following simple key:

Plants with leaves
    1. On *Juniperus* or *Cupressus* .... *Phoradendron densum*
    2. On *Abies concolor* .... *P. pauciflorum*

Plants without leaves
    1. On *Juniperus* .... *P. juniperinum*
    2. On *Libocedrus* .... *P. libocedri*

Cypress-Juniper Mistletoe
"Dense" Mistletoe
Phoradendron densum

Hosts—*Phoradendron densum* infects several species of cypress and juniper in the West.

Distribution and damage—This mistletoe is widespread throughout certain areas of California. Its occurrence on cypress ranges along the Pacific Coast from the mountains of northwestern California southward to Marin County. Inland, it ranges from Butte County, CA, northward along the western slope of the Sierra Nevada and into the Cascade Range in southern Oregon. This mistletoe is also found on cypress in central Arizona.

On juniper, the mistletoe extends from Baja California and Arizona northward along the eastern slope of the Sierra Nevada and southern Cascades. Along the California coast, it ranges from San Diego to Monterey County.

Many plants may occur on and damage individual trees. But losses to forests from this particular mistletoe appear minimal.

Field identification—This is the only leafy mistletoe on cypress or juniper. Clusters of greenish mistletoe foliage occur on branches throughout the host crown. The shoots bear narrow leaves that are usually about 2 to 5 mm wide and 12 to 20 mm long (fig. 5-5a,b).

White Fir Mistletoe
Phoradendron pauciflorum

Hosts—White fir is the only host.

Distribution and damage—White fir growing in the Sierra Nevada from Placer County southward and in the mountains of southern California is the host of this parasite. Curiously, red fir is not attacked, even in areas where this tree grows in mixed stands with white fir. It also occurs in the Santa Catalina Mountains of Arizona and the Sierra San Pedro Martir in Baja California, Mexico.

This mistletoe is, for the most part, a serious parasite of only larger and older trees. Many years are required for populations to build up and become damaging to white fir. In some instances, the parasite becomes so dense that tree tops and sometimes entire trees are weakened and die or are attacked and killed by bark beetles.

Figure 5-5—
The leafy plant growing on the branch of western juniper is the dense mistletoe, Phoradendron densum *(**a**). Western juniper often becomes severely infected by the dense mistletoe (**b**).*

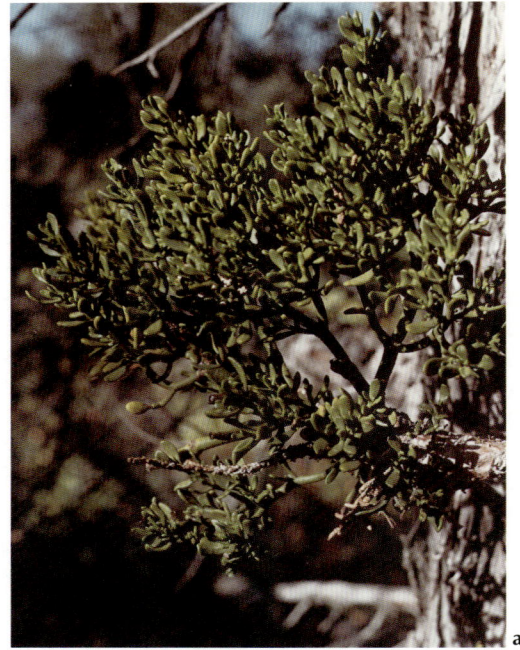

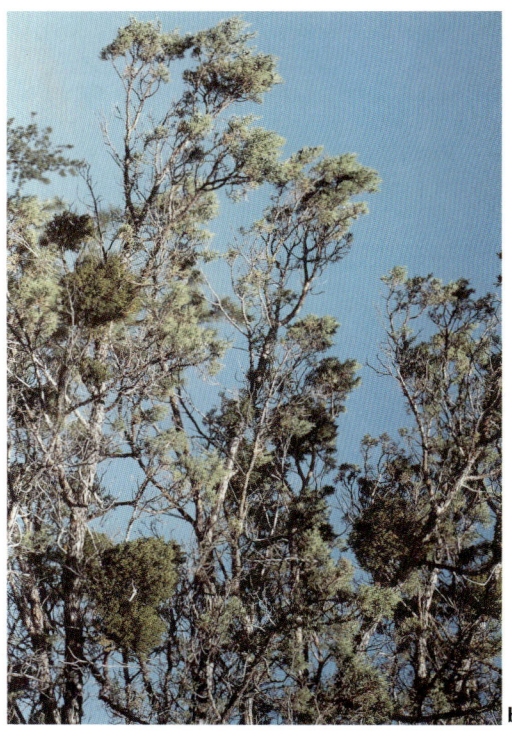

Another important effect is that heavily infected trees produce no cones.

Field identification—This is the only leafy mistletoe on white fir. This mistletoe is often observed in the tops of the tallest trees in the stand. Large clumps of foliage may grow along the trunk of the tree for 20 to 30 feet (6 to 9 m) down from the top (fig. 5-4). Often the tree foliage in this zone is nearly completely replaced by mistletoe foliage. Spike tops are also common in white fir stands infected with this parasite. The dead mistletoe shoots remain attached to the dead top and branches for some years after death. The leaves are dark green, narrow, and about 5 to 8 mm wide and 15 to 30 mm long.

Juniper Mistletoe
Phoradendron juniperinum

Hosts—Several species of juniper are hosts, but western juniper is by far the most common host.

Distribution and damage—Along the Pacific Coast, this mistletoe ranges from the eastern slope of the southern Cascade Range in central Oregon through the upper elevations of the Sierra Nevada, and south into the San Bernardino Mountains of southern California. Elsewhere in the western United States, it extends from northern Utah into northern Mexico. Although this mistletoe builds up to high populations on some trees, the damage it causes to stands appears to be negligible.

Field identification—This is the only leafless mistletoe on junipers (fig. 5-2). *P. juniperinum* appears as round clumps of green to yellowish shoots, usually in the tops of trees. The most distinctive characteristic that distinguishes it from *P. densum,* which also grows on junipers, is the absence of leaves. The leaves on this particular species are reduced to inconspicuous scales less than 3 mm long. Berries are light pink.

Incense-Cedar Mistletoe
Phoradendron libocedri

Hosts—Incense-cedar is the only host.

Distribution and damage—Incense-cedar mistletoe is found in southern Oregon, on the western slope of the Sierra Nevada, in the mountains of southern California, and in the Sierra San Pedro Martir in Baja California. For the most part, this mistletoe causes negligible damage to its host. On older trees, however, it occasionally builds up to high populations. It may weaken a tree, but rarely kills it.

Field identification—This species is the only mistletoe on incense-cedar. Round, usually pendant, green clumps of mistletoe shoots in the crowns of incense-cedar identify this organism (fig. 5-1). The mistletoe is sometimes confused with the dense, deformed branches caused by incense-cedar rust (see Chap. 4). Like another mistletoe that occurs on juniper, the leaves are inconspicuous scales about 3 mm long. This mistletoe occasionally infects tree trunks and causes some swelling, but this occurs only in cases in which the root system of the parasite has been in the trunk for many years. The berries are light pink (fig. 5-3).

DWARF MISTLETOES*

Unlike the true mistletoes, dwarf mistletoes depend almost entirely on food produced by the host; they photosynthesize little material for themselves.

The aerial shoot system, therefore, functions mainly for reproduction. Small, inconspicuous flowers are produced in the axils of the shoot segment (fig. 5-6). Flowers are pollinated by both insects and wind. Short stalks bear fruits that are about 3 mm long when ripe (fig. 5-7).

Unlike the true mistletoes, dwarf mistletoes are only rarely disseminated by birds, but depend on an explosive mechanism for spread. During maturation the fruits swell with water and build up considerable hydraulic pressure. At maturity the seeds, usually one per fruit, are explosively discharged by the water pressure in the fruit. Discharged seeds may travel horizontally for 30 to 40 feet (9 to 12 m). With the aid of the wind, seeds discharged from the tops of trees may travel as far as 100 feet (30 m) or more.

Like those of the true mistletoes, the seeds of dwarf mistletoes are sticky. They initially adhere to the foliage of surrounding branches and trees (fig. 5-8). During rains, the seeds swell with water, become slippery, and wash down on and adhere to host branches, where they germinate and infect the host. The root system of dwarf mistletoe penetrates and grows within the tree branch in much the same way as do true mistletoes.

Trees respond in several ways to infection by dwarf mistletoe. Usually a localized swelling of the branch occurs (fig. 5-9). Occasionally pronounced swelling of the main stem of a tree occurs as a result of the parasite infecting the trunk directly or by growing into the trunk from an infected branch. With time these swellings may grow to a size of twice the normal diameter of the tree trunk. To compound the problem in firs and hemlocks, decay fungi often enter bark cracks and openings at the site of swelling, causing heart rot (fig. 5-10).

---

*The genus of dwarf mistletoe was revised, and many of the species names used reflect changes in the names of the previously known dwarf mistletoes in western North America (Hawksworth and Wiens 1972; Hawksworth, Wiens, and Nickrent 1991).

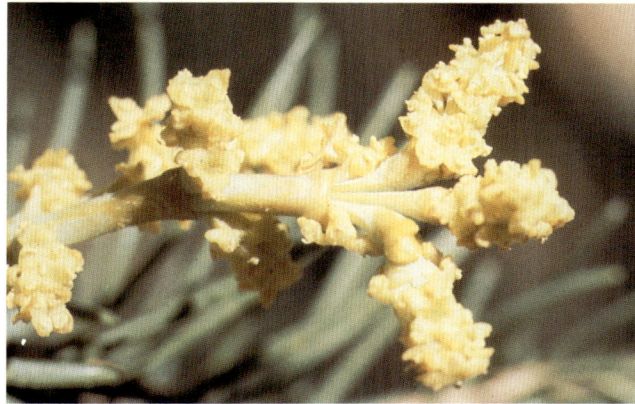

Figure 5-6—*Shoot from male plant of red fir dwarf mistletoe (Arceuthobium abietinum f. sp. magnificae) bearing mature flowers.*

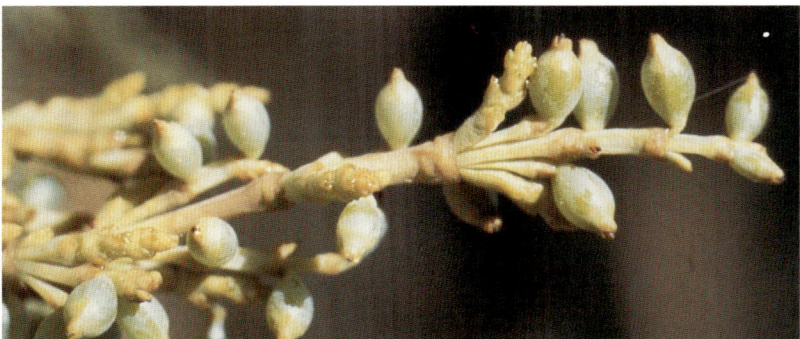

Figure 5-7—*Shoot from female plant of red fir dwarf mistletoe bearing mature fruit.*

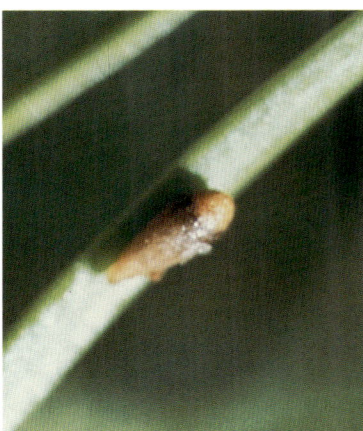

Figure 5-8—*Seed of white fir dwarf mistletoe (Arceuthobium abietinum f. sp. concoloris) adhering to needles of white fir.*

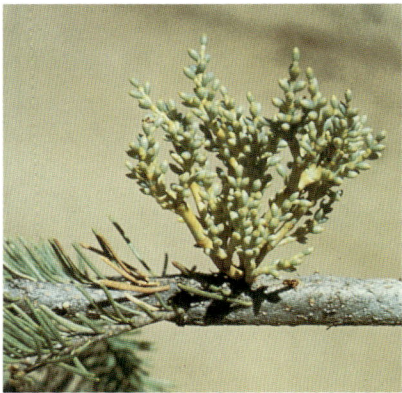

Figure 5-9—*A white fir dwarf mistletoe plant arising from the infected, swollen part of a branch of white fir.*

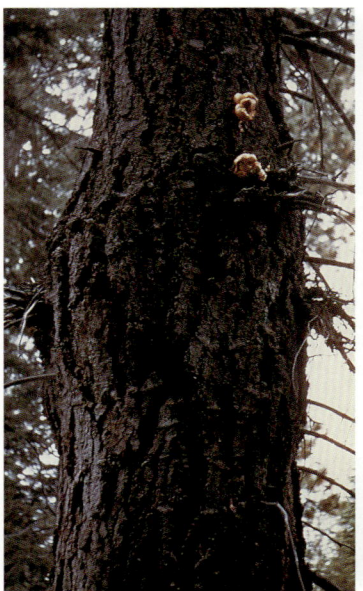

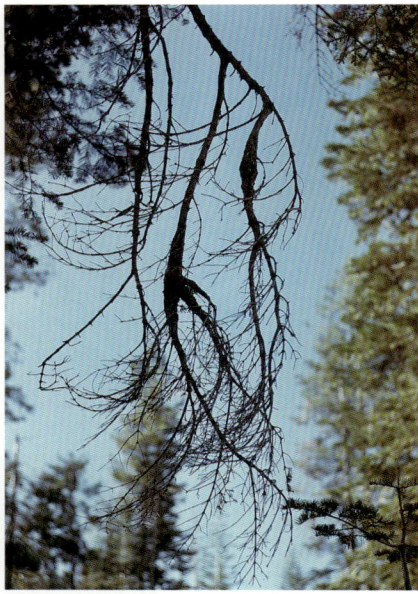

Figure 5-10—*Decayed bole swelling on white fir caused by white fir dwarf mistletoe. Note fruiting body of the decay fungus* (Pholiota adiposa) *growing out of the mistletoe-infected portion of the stem.*

Figure 5-11—*Characteristically open, fan-shaped brooms on white fir are caused by white fir dwarf mistletoe.*

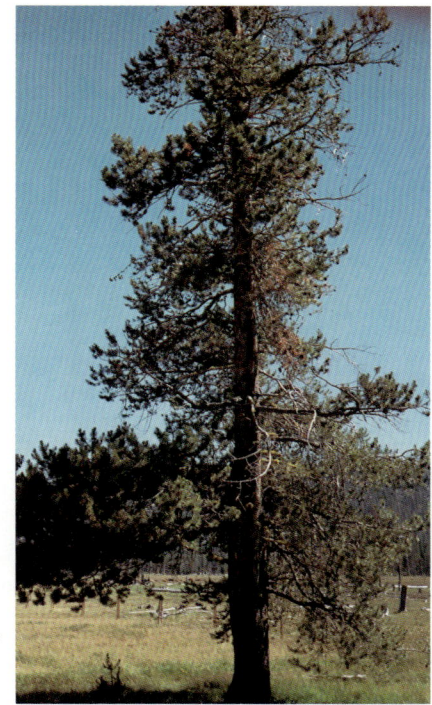

Figure 5-12—*Large, conspicuous brooms are common on lodgepole pines infected by the dwarf mistletoe* (Arceuthobium americanum).

Frequently these decaying trees break at the swelling, causing loss of timber and presenting a hazard in recreational and high-use areas.

With most dwarf mistletoe species, host branches react to infection by producing what is commonly known as a witches-broom or broom. A broom is an abnormal proliferation of many small twigs on a branch that appear as a clustered mass of twigs and foliage. Brooms vary in appearance from ball-shaped to loose fan-shaped structures. Some brooms remain small (fig. 5-11), whereas others may comprise the bulk of the foliage on a tree (fig. 5-12).

Most species of dwarf mistletoe are host-specific and occur on only one species of tree. Others may occur on two or three different species of conifers. Only a few cross infect from one genus of conifer to another. When they do, they usually spread from the primary host to secondary hosts in stands in which both hosts are growing close to one another. As a result of their host specificity, the dwarf mistletoes of the western United States can best be distinguished from one another on the basis of host species and host distribution.

DESCRIPTIVE KEY

Note: This key is based on the *main* hosts of the dwarf mistletoe in a particular area. Most species will sometimes attack other associated trees.

A^1	On pines	B
B^1	On pinyons	*Arceuthobium divaricatum*
B^2	On 2 & 3 needle pines	C
C^1	On lodgepole pine	*A. americanum*
C^2	On shore pine, San Juan Islands, Wash.	*A. tsugense* subsp. *tsugense*
C^3	On ponderosa, Jeffrey, or Coulter pine	*A. campylopodum*
C^4	On Digger pine	*A. occidentale*
C^5	On knobcone pine (NW California and SW Oregon)	*A. siskiyouense*
C^6	On Monterey or bishop pines	*A. littorum*
B^3	On 5-needle pines	D
D^1	On limber or whitebark pines	*A. cyanocarpum*
D^2	On sugar pine	*A. californicum*
D^3	On western white pine	E
E^1	NW California and SW Oregon.	*A. monticolum*
E^2	Sierra Nevada and Cascades, associated with infected mountain hemlock	*A. tsugense* subsp. *mertensianae*
A^2	On firs	F
F^1	On white fir or grand fir	*A. abietinum* f. sp. *concoloris*
F^2	On red fir	*A. abietinum* f. sp. *magnificae*
F^3	On noble or Pacific silver fir	*A. tsugense**

A³ On hemlocks .... G
G¹ On mountain hemlock .... *A. tsugense* subsp. *mertensianae*
G² On western hemlock .... *A. tsugense* subsp. *tsugense*
A⁴ On Douglas-fir .... *A. douglasii*
A⁵ On western larch. .... *A. laricis*

True Fir Dwarf Mistletoe
***Arceuthobium abietinum* (f. sp. *concoloris*)—white fir & grand fir; (f. sp. *magnificae*)—red fir**

Hosts—*Arceuthobium abietinum* has two specialized host forms. These forms, although identical in appearance, are host-specific—one infecting only red fir (f. sp. *magnificae*) and the other infecting only white fir and grand fir (f. sp. *concoloris*). The white fir—grand fir form has never been found on red fir and rarely infects sugar pine in the Sierra Nevada and Brewer spruce in southern Oregon.

Distribution and damage—Fir dwarf mistletoes are common and widespread on their hosts through their range in the central and southern Cascades (from southern Washington southward through the Sierra Nevada to the mountains of southern California). They also occur in the coastal mountains of northern California and southern Oregon, and in some areas extending almost down to sea level on grand fir in Mendocino County. In California about 30 percent of the white fir stands and about 50 percent of the red fir stands are infested with this parasite. As a result of its widespread distribution, dwarf mistletoe constitutes one of the most serious forest disease problems in the management of true firs.

Field identification—This is the only leafless mistletoe on white fir. The presence of dwarf mistletoe plants and fusiform branch swellings are sure signs of infection (fig. 5-9). One of the best indicators of infection in fir stands is the presence of branch flagging. Branches infected by dwarf mistletoe are commonly attacked and killed by a canker fungus, *Cytospora abietis*, and flagging results (chap. 3, fig. 3-6). The brick-red flagged branches are most conspicuous in late spring and summer when the foliage on the killed branch begins to dry. Later in the fall the dead foliage turns more gray brown in color. Large swellings as a result of invasion of the tree trunk by the parasite are common on large, old firs (fig. 5-10). These swellings are often very pronounced and may reach a diameter of twice the normal size of the trunk. Some brooming occurs on older infected

---

* Both subspecies of *A. tsugense* attack these firs. Subspecies *tsugense* is the most common of them, and it parasitizes associated western hemlock, but not mountain hemlock. Subspecies *mertensianae* is rather rare on these firs but is found in higher parts of the Oregon Cascade Range; it will parasitize associated mountain hemlock but not western hemlock.

branches but is not conspicuous (fig. 5-11). Brooms caused by fir broom rust (see chapter 4) also occur on firs in the western United States and could be confused with those caused by dwarf mistletoe. Shoots are green to yellow-green, usually 4 to 6 inches (10 to 15 cm) high.

Lodgepole Pine Dwarf Mistletoe
Arceuthobium americanum

Hosts—Lodgepole pine (*Pinus contorta* var. *murrayana* in California and Oregon and var. *latifolia* in Oregon and Washington) are the common hosts for this dwarf mistletoe, although it has been found rarely on ponderosa pine.

Distribution and damage—*Arceuthobium americanum* has the widest range of any North American dwarf mistletoe, mainly because of the wide range of its principal host. It occurs throughout the western United States and Canada. On the Pacific Coast it occurs on lodgepole pine in the Cascade Range and the Sierra Nevada. It has not been found on shore pine (*P. contorta* var. *contorta*) or Bolander pine (*P. contorta* var. *bolanderi*) along the coast.

Forest disease surveys indicate that nearly 30 percent of the lodgepole pine stands in California are infested with this parasite. Where it occurs it is damaging and causes considerable growth reduction and mortality to lodgepole pine.

Field identification—This is the only common mistletoe on lodgepole pine. Pronounced brooming of trees is the most conspicuous symptom of infection (fig. 5-12). Brooms on older, heavily infected trees often make up nearly the entire live crown. The presence of dwarf mistletoe plants and some fusiform swelling of branches also indicate infection. Shoots are greenish, usually 2 to 3 inches (5 to 8 cm) high.

Sugar Pine Dwarf Mistletoe
Arceuthobium californicum

Hosts—The principal host of this mistletoe is sugar pine. It occurs rarely on western white pine when it grows near infected sugar pines.

Distribution and damage—*Arceuthobium californicum* is found from the Mt. Shasta area south through the Coast Range in northern California to Lake County and in the Sierra Nevada to southern California (San Gabriel, San Bernardino, San Jacinto, and Cuyamaca Mountains). It apparently occurred in Oregon south of Crater Lake earlier in this century, but not now.

Although this mistletoe occurs essentially throughout the natural range of sugar pine in California, it is not as common as dwarf mistletoes on other species. Forest disease surveys have shown that about 20 percent of the forest stands containing sugar pine are

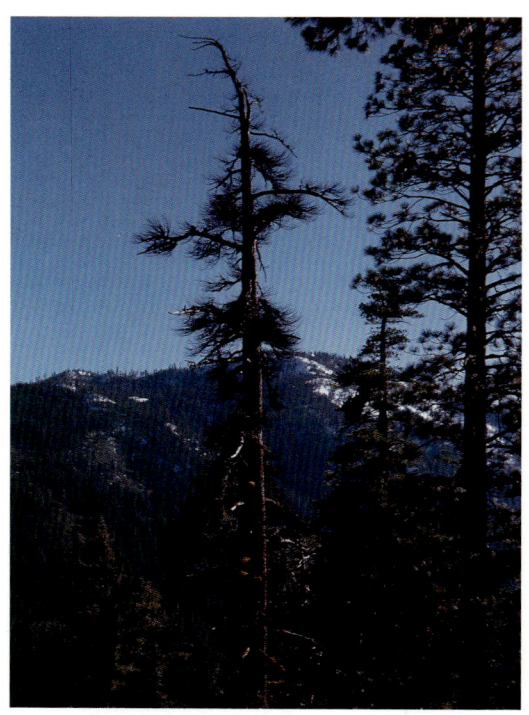

Figure 5-13—
Sugar pine dwarf mistletoe (Arceuthobium californicum) often forms large brooms on infected sugar pine.

infested with this parasite. The frequency of dwarf mistletoe on sugar pine is probably lower than on other host species because sugar pine rarely forms pure stands. Sugar pine occurs in mixture with other conifer species but seldom comprises more than 50 percent of a stand. This mixed-stand situation undoubtedly limits the spread of the parasite under natural forest conditions.

Where sugar pine is infected, heavy damage can occur. Numerous infections may develop and large brooms on older trees are common. Heavy infection severely reduces growth. Weakened trees are also often attacked and killed by bark beetles.

Field identification—This is the only dwarf mistletoe commonly found on sugar pine. Large compact brooms in the crowns of older trees are the best symptoms of infection (fig. 5-13). Numerous individual fusiform branch swellings and the presence of aerial shoots of the parasite are also easily recognized symptoms and signs of infection. Shoots are yellow to green, usually 3 to 4 inches (5 to 8 cm) high.

Western Dwarf Mistletoe
Arceuthobium campylopodum

Hosts—Western dwarf mistletoe is found on ponderosa pine, Jeffrey pine, knobcone pine, and Coulter pine. It occasionally occurs on Digger pine associated with infected ponderosa pine in the higher elevations, usually over 4,500 feet (1,372 m) in the southern Sierra Nevada (Fresno, Kern, and Tulare Counties).

Distribution and damage—*Arceuthobium campylopodum* ranges throughout the ponderosa pine forests of western North America from Washington and Idaho, through Oregon and California, to northern Baja California, Mexico. In Washington it occurs only east of the Cascade Crest. In Oregon it is common east of the Cascade Crest, and in southern part of the state (Josephine, Jackson, and Klamath Counties); it was apparently once common in the Willamette Valley but is very rare there now. In California it is common in the coastal mountains south to Lake County and in the southern Cascades and Sierras to southern California (to San Diego County), but not in the South Coast ranges where a related species *(A. occidentale)* replaces it on ponderosa pine and other pines.

The western dwarf mistletoe is one of the most damaging forest pests in the western United States. Many commercial pine stands there have been killed or suffered reduced growth because of it (fig. 5-14a). Jeffrey pine is considered to be more susceptible to this parasite than ponderosa pine, but both species are heavily attacked. Coulter and Jeffrey pines in southern California suffer heavy mortality and are among the most seriously damaged species.

Field identification—This is the only common mistletoe on ponderosa pine or Jeffrey pine in the Pacific Coast States (except in the south Coast Ranges of California). The fusiform branch swellings and aerial shoots of the plant are conspicuous indications of infection (fig. 5-14b). Brooms may form, and on larger trees, they become well developed and are easily observed (fig. 5-14c). Swelling as a result of trunk infection is not pronounced as that in true firs. But, in some cases, old trunk infections result in open, pitch-infiltrated, diamond-shaped bole cankers. Shoots are green to yellow, usually 4 to 5 inches (10 to 13 cm) high.

Limber Pine Dwarf Mistletoe
Arceuthobium cyanocarpum

Hosts—*Arceuthobium cyanocarpum* mainly occurs on limber or whitebark pines, rarely on foxtail or western white pines.

Distribution and damage—*Arceuthobium cyanocarpum* is most common in the Great Basin and Rocky Mountain regions. In the far western United States, it occurs only locally: it is known in only one area in Oregon (west of Bend), and in two locations in northern California (near Mt. Shasta and in the Warner Mountains). It is found on a number of areas on the east side of the Sierra Nevada and in the desert ranges in Mono and Inyo Counties and in the San Bernardino and San Jacinto mountains in southern California.

Figure 5-14—*Young Jeffrey pines are often severely stunted and deformed by western dwarf mistletoe* (Arceuthobium campylopodum) *(**a**). The male plants of western dwarf mistletoe are usually more orange than the female plants (**b**). Conspicuous brooms are often observed in the crowns of large trees infected by western dwarf mistletoe (**c**).*

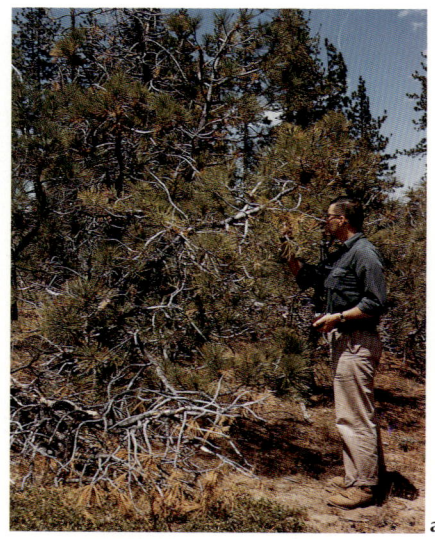

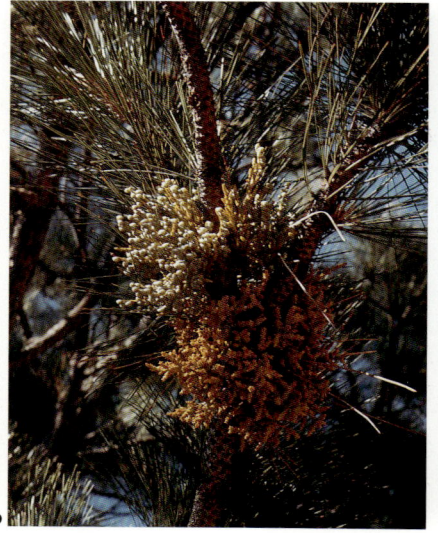

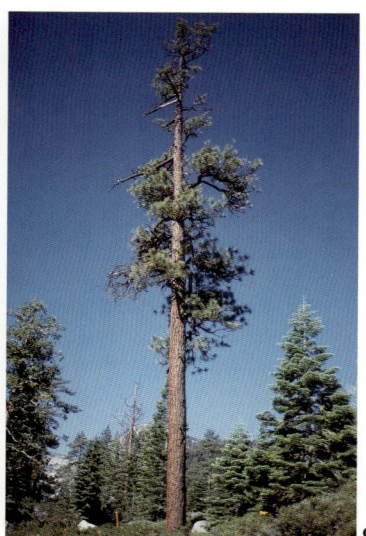

Infected trees are often severely damaged and deformed and many of them die (fig. 5-15).

Field identification—*A. cyanocarpum* is the only common mistletoe on limber and whitebark pines. Infected trees bear numerous infections, and the parasite is easily recognized by the presence of numerous small, densely clustered shoots. Brooms are formed, but are typically small and compact. Trees die in infested stands to such

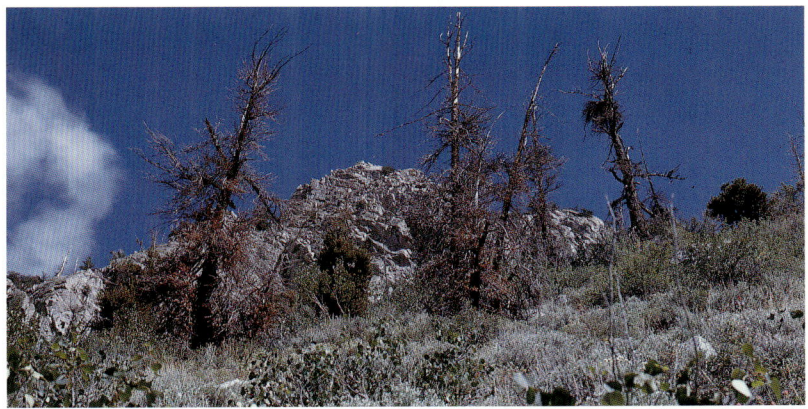

Figure 5-15—*Dying limber pine in California heavily infected by limber pine dwarf mistletoe (*Arceuthobium cyanocarpum*)*

an extent that "ghost forests" result. Shoots are yellow green, usually 1 to 2 inches (3 to 5 cm) high.

Pinyon Dwarf Mistletoe
Arceuthobium divaricatum

Hosts—Singleleaf pinyon is the common host; also found on Parry pinyon in northern Baja California and reported on this host in San Diego County, CA.

Distribution and damage—*Arceuthobium divaricatum* infects several species of pinyons in the Rocky Mountains, the southwestern United States, and Baja California, Mexico. In California it occurs on the east side of the Sierra Nevada (from Alpine County south), in the Mohave Desert mountain ranges, and in the southern mountains (Ventura to San Diego Counties). Damage is usually not severe even when trees are heavily infected. Tree mortality is slight, although growth is reduced.

Field identification—This is the only mistletoe in pinyons. Heavily infected trees often bear hundreds of individual branch infections. Broom formation, however, is not conspicuous. Shoots are brown, usually 3 to 4 inches (8 to 10 cm) high (fig. 5-16).

Douglas-Fir Dwarf Mistletoe
Arceuthobium douglasii

Hosts—The principal host is Douglas-fir, but *Arceuthobium douglasii* rarely occurs on several species of true fir and spruce in association with infected Douglas-fir.

Distribution and damage—*A. douglasii* occurs on Douglas-fir in Washington and most of Oregon only east of the crest of the Cas-

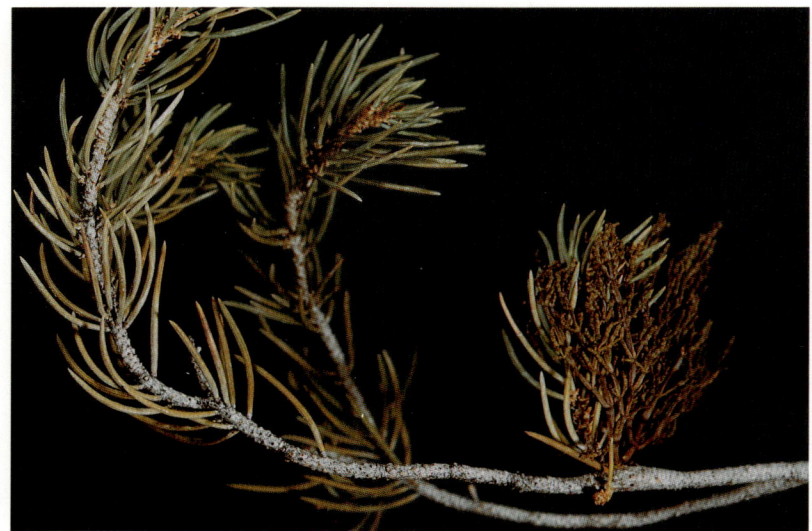

Figure 5-16—*Branches of pinyon pine infected by pinyon dwarf mistletoe* (Arceuthobium divaricatum) *seldom develop into brooms.*

cades. Elsewhere, it occurs on Douglas-fir from southern British Columbia to central Mexico. Only in southwestern Oregon and California does it occur in the coastal mountains (south to Trinity and Tehama Counties). It is less common in the Cascade Range and Sierra Nevadas and has been found south to Plumas County.

Douglas-fir is severely damaged by this parasite. Heavily infected trees are weakened, deformed, and often killed. Because Douglas-fir often grows in pure stands or is the predominant species, damage to commercial forests by this mistletoe is often widespread.

Field identification—This is the only mistletoe on Douglas-fir. Huge brooms are common on older infected trees (fig. 5-17) and are nearly certain indication of infection by dwarf mistletoe. Young infected trees may be stunted and deformed. The mistletoe plant itself is very small and inconspicuous. The aerial shoots often arise from along infected branches of a broom or from the spindle-shaped localized infections. Shoots are green, usually only about 1 inch (3 cm) high (fig. 5-18).

Larch Dwarf Mistletoe
Arceuthobium laricis

Hosts—Western larch is the principal host for this species. Several other conifers are sometimes infected when they grow in association with infected larch.

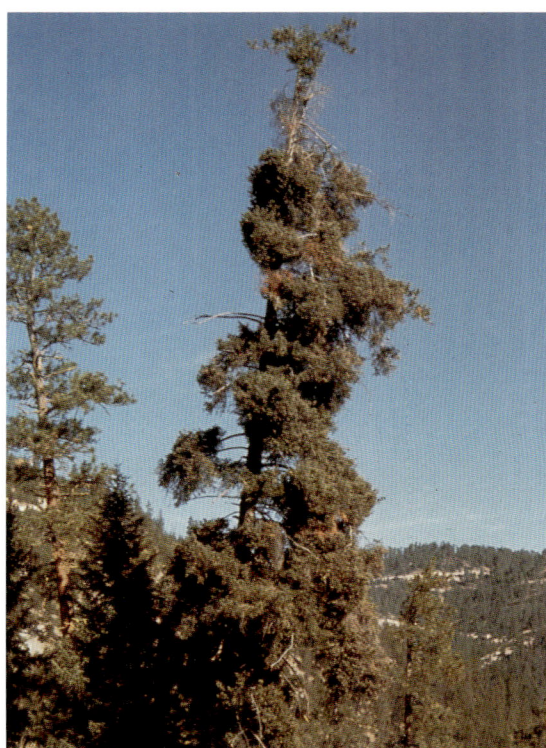

Figure 5-17—*Massive, tight brooms develop on Douglas-fir as a result of infection by Douglas-fir dwarf mistletoe* (Arceuthobium douglasii).

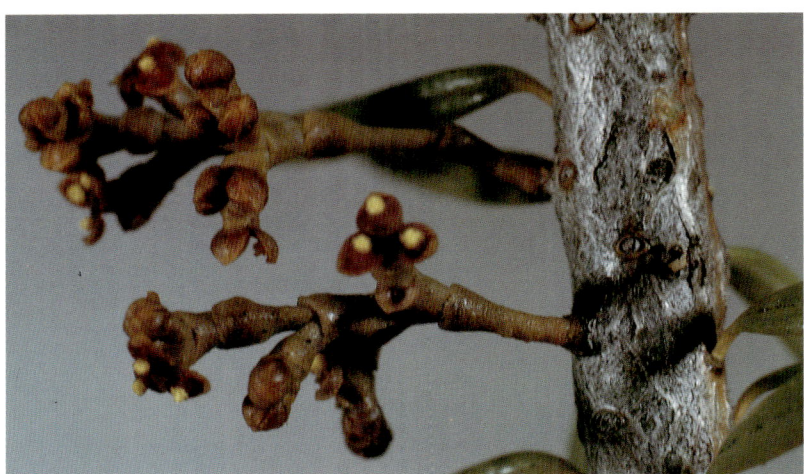

Figure 5-18—*Small, inconspicuous plants are produced by Douglas-fir dwarf mistletoe. (Note male shoots with mature male flowers).*

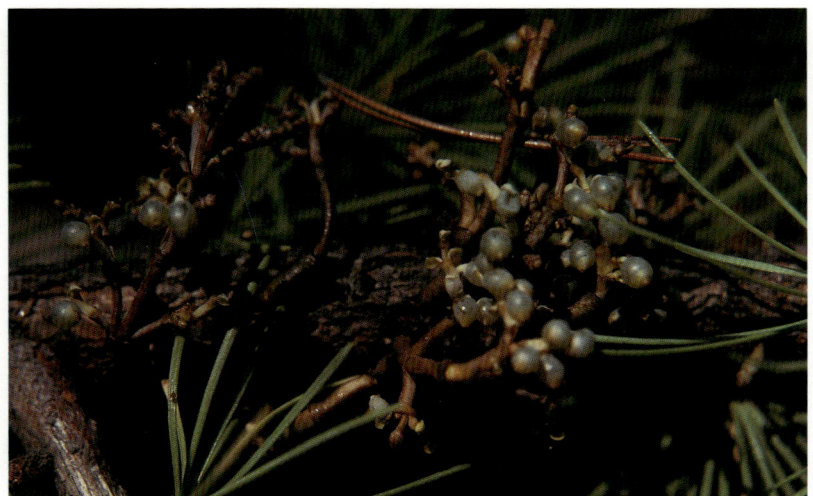

Figure 5-19—*Fruit of larch dwarf mistletoe (*Arceuthobium laricis*) are produced on short, dark shoots.*

Distribution and damage—In general, larch dwarf mistletoe occurs throughout the range of western larch. It is found east of the Cascade Range in Oregon and in Washington but does not occur in California. Western larch suffers severe damage from larch dwarf mistletoe. A high proportion of larch stands are badly infested, and heavy mortality and growth loss are common.

Field identification—*A. laricis* is the only mistletoe on western larch. Pronounced brooming of older trees is the most conspicuous symptom of infection. Badly infected trees have literally dozens of brooms; these are particularly noticeable in fall and winter after the deciduous foliage of larch has been shed. Shoots are purple or green, usually 2 to 3 inches (5 to 8 cm) high (fig. 5-19).

Coastal Dwarf Mistletoe
Arceuthobium littorum

Hosts—Monterey and bishop pines are the main hosts of coastal dwarf mistletoe. Bolander pine is a rare host in Mendocino County, CA.

Distribution and damage—*Arceuthobium littorum* has a limited range from Mendocino to San Luis Obispo Counties. It occurs only at relatively low elevations and within about 5 miles of the Pacific Ocean. The mistletoe causes extensive brooming and distortion of its hosts but relatively little mortality.

Field identification—*A. littorum* is the only mistletoe in natural stands of Monterey or bishop pines. It forms conspicuous fusiform swellings. Shoots are dark yellow to brown, usually 5 to 6 inches (13 to 15 cm) high.

Western White Pine Dwarf Mistletoe
Arceuthobium monticolum

Hosts—Essentially restricted to western white pine, rare on associated sugar pine.

Distribution and damage—This local species occurs only in the Siskiyou Mountains of northwestern California (Del Norte and western Siskiyou Counties) and the Klamath Mountains in adjacent southwestern Oregon (Coos, Curry, and Josephine Counties).

Field identification—This is the main mistletoe on western white pine in the Siskiyou and Klamath Mountains. Trees are usually heavily infected with many fusiform branch infections (fig. 5-20). Brooming and tree mortality are limited. Shoots are dark brown, usually 3 to 4 inches (8 to 10 cm) high.

Digger Pine Dwarf Mistletoe
Arceuthobium occidentale

Hosts—Digger pine is by far the main host, but this mistletoe will sometimes occur on associated knobcone and Coulter pines. In the southern Coastal Range, it occurs on ponderosa, Coulter, and Jeffrey pines.

Distribution and damage—This mistletoe occurs on Digger pine essentially throughout the range of this tree. It also occurs on Coulter pine or knobcone pine when these trees are associated with infected Digger pine; it very rarely occurs on associated ponderosa pine.

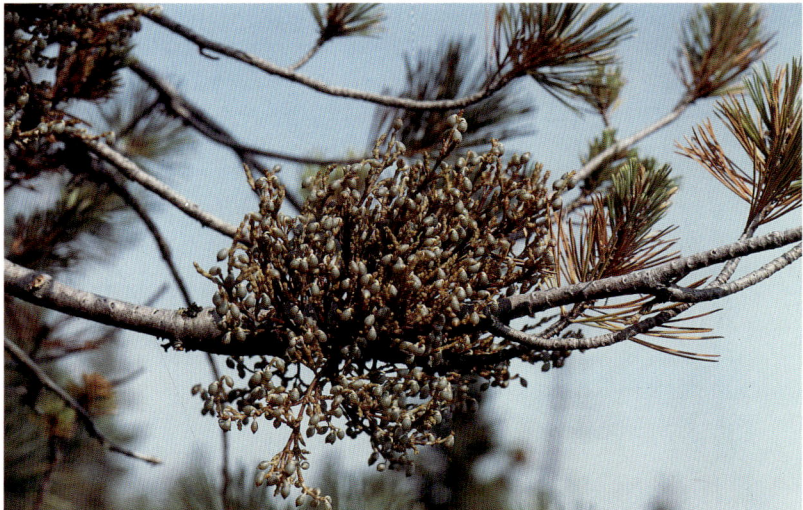

Figure 5-20—*Robust female plants of western white pine dwarf mistletoe* (Arceuthobium monticolum) *on western white pine often produce abundant shoots and fruit.*

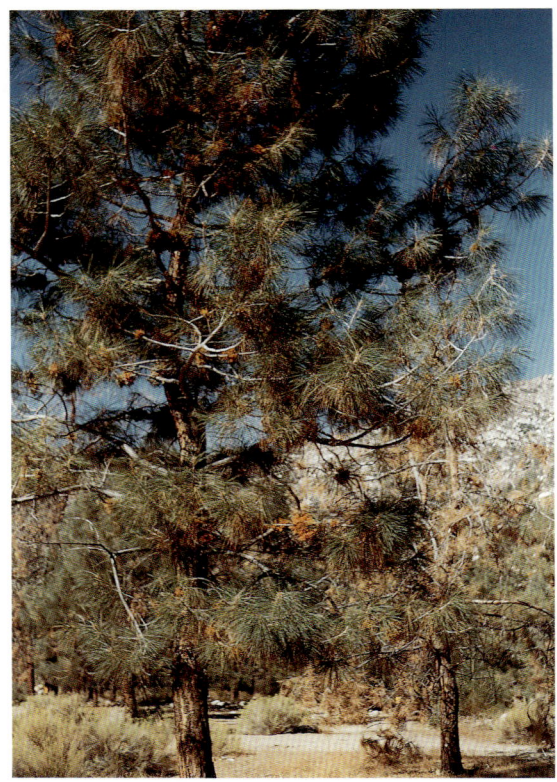

Figure 5-21—*Digger pine often become heavily infected with large clumps of Digger pine dwarf mistletoe* (Arceuthobium occidentale) *but few brooms develop.*

Digger pine is severely damaged: trees are reduced in growth, deformed, and often killed. Hundreds of individual infections may occur on trees over a period of just several years, and the upward spread of the parasite on this host species is known to be very rapid and equal to the growth in height of even vigorous trees.

Field identification—Digger pine dwarf mistletoe is the only mistletoe on Digger pine. The numerous dwarf mistletoe plants and fusiform swollen branches are probably the best signs and symptoms of infection (fig. 5-21). Because of the rapid rate of buildup and upward spread of this parasite, infections may be seen throughout the crowns of heavily infected trees. Although some brooms are formed, brooms never become as well developed as those caused by most dwarf mistletoes in pines. Shoots are yellowish, usually 4 to 5 inches (10 to 13 cm) high.

Knobcone Pine Dwarf Mistletoe
Arceuthobium siskiyouense

Hosts—The main host is knobcone pine, but associated ponderosa pine and Jeffrey pines are sometimes rarely infected.

Distribution and damage—Knobcone pine dwarf mistletoe is a local species confined to the Siskiyou Mountains in northwestern California (Del Norte and western Siskiyou Counties) and the Klamath Mountains in adjacent southwestern Oregon (Curry and Josephine Counties). The mistletoe does not form witches-brooms, but older infected branches become quite swollen. Infection is often heavy, and trees may bear hundreds of infections. Mortality is often severe, particularly in dense stands.

Field identification—Knobcone pine dwarf mistletoe is the only common mistletoe on knobcone pine in the Siskiyou and Klamath Mountain Ranges. Fusiform swellings with abundant dwarf mistletoe shoots are the best indicators of infection. Shoots are yellow to brown, usually 2 to 3 inches (5 to 8 cm) high.

Western Hemlock Dwarf Mistletoe
Arceuthobium tsugense subsp. *tsugense*

Hosts—Western hemlock dwarf mistletoe attacks mainly western hemlock, but it also parasitizes associated noble fir in Oregon and Pacific silver fir in Oregon and Washington. Associated mountain hemlock is very rarely infected. A local race of this mistletoe is essentially confined to shore pine on Orcas Island, WA, and in coastal British Columbia.

Distribution and damage—This mistletoe occurs on western hemlock along the Pacific Coast from southeastern Alaska (near Haines) to northern California (Humboldt County). It is common in the Oregon and Washington Coast and Cascade Ranges but rare in California. Damage by this mistletoe in western hemlock is most severe in old-growth stands, but young stands are also damaged in some areas. Severe growth loss, deformation, and mortality result from heavy infection.

Field identification—This is the only mistletoe on western hemlock. Brooming of older trees is the most noticeable symptom of infection. Brooms are often large and abundant. Smaller trees are often severely stunted. Aerial shoots of the plant are not always formed, particularly under the densely shaded conditions of the coastal forests. Only under open growing conditions or in the tops of trees does the parasite produce many aerial shoots. Spindle-shaped branch swellings also are indicative of infection. Shoots are greenish, usually 2 to 3 inches (5 to 8 cm) high.

Mountain Hemlock Dwarf Mistletoe
Arceuthobium tsugense subsp. *mertensianae*

Hosts—The main host of *Arceuthobium tsugense* subsp. *mertensianae* is mountain hemlock, but associated western white pines are also commonly infected. In the Oregon Cascades, the

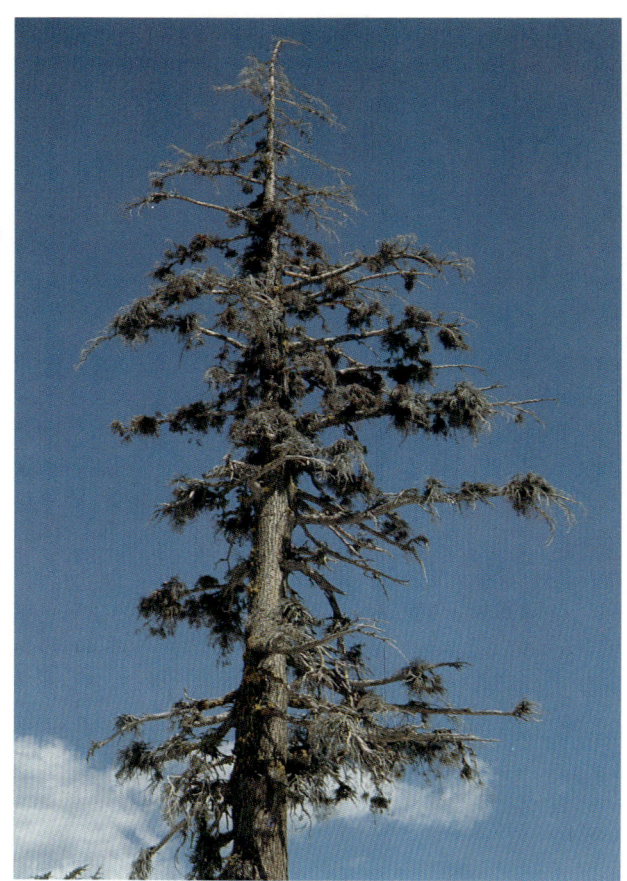

Figure 5-22— *Large mountain hemlock are often killed by mountain hemlock dwarf mistletoe (Arceuthobium tsugense subsp. mertensianae).* Note the numerous compact brooms formed on branches.

mistletoe also attacks noble fir, Pacific silver fir, subalpine fir, and white bark pine, but not western hemlock.

Distribution and damage—This mistletoe occurs in the higher elevations of the Cascade Range from central Oregon (Linn County) to the central Sierra Nevada (Alpine County). It causes severe broom formation, growth loss, and mortality in mountain hemlock and western white pine (fig. 5-22).

Field identification—This is the only mistletoe on mountain hemlock; associated western white pines are usually heavily infected as well. Marked witches-broom formation and heavy tree mortality characterize this species. Shoots are greenish, usually 2 to 3 inches (5 to 8 cm) high.

SELECTED REFERENCES

Gill, Lake S.; Hawksworth, Frank G. 1961. The mistletoes: a literature review. Tech. Bull. 1241, Washington, DC: U.S. Department of Agriculture. 87 p.

Hawksworth, Frank G. 1961. Dwarf mistletoe of ponderosa pine in the Southwest. Tech. Bull. 1246. Washington, DC: U.S. Department of Agriculture. 112 p.

Hawksworth, Frank G.; Wiens, Delbert. 1972. Biology and classification of the dwarf mistletoes (*Arceuthobium*). Agric. Handb. 401. Washington, DC: U.S. Department of Agriculture. 234 p.

Hawksworth, Frank G.; Wiens, Delbert; Nickrent, Daniel L. 1993. New western taxa of Arceuthobium (Viscaceae). Madrono (in press).

Kuijt, Job. 1955. Dwarf mistletoes. Botanical Review 21:569–627.

Scharpf, Robert F. 1964. Dwarf mistletoe on true firs in California. Forest Pest Leafl. 89. Washington, DC: U.S. Department of Agriculture. 7 p.

Scharpf, Robert F.; Hawksworth, Frank G. 1968. Dwarf mistletoe on sugar pine. Forest Pest Leafl. 113. Washington, DC: U.S. Department of Agriculture. 4 p.

Scharpf, Robert F.; Parmeter, J.R., Jr. 1967. The biology and pathology of dwarf mistletoe, *Arceuthobium campylopodum* f. *abietinum* parasitizing true firs (*Abies* ssp.) in California. Tech. Bull. 1362. Washington, DC: U.S. Department of Agriculture. 42 p.

Walters, James. 1976. A guide to disease of southwestern conifers. Bulletin R3-78-9. Albuquerque, NM: U.S. Department of Agriculture, Forest Service, Southwestern Region.

Wiens, Delbert. 1964. Revision of the acataphyllous species of *Phoradendron*. Britonnia 16(1):11–54.

CHAPTER 6   Root Diseases

Richard S. Smith, Jr.
Principal Plant Pathologist, formerly with the Pacific Southwest Forest and Range Experiment Station and the California Region; now with Forest Insect and Disease Research, Forest Service, U.S. Department of Agriculture, Washington, DC.

INTRODUCTION

Root diseases are becoming increasingly more important in the forests of the western United States. Each year more areas of root disease infestation and greater numbers of infected trees are detected because of increased awareness, more intensive surveys, and better diagnostic techniques. In many areas, past forest management practices have increased the incidence and severity of root diseases, and unless control measures are taken, they will continue to do so in the future.

The major root diseases in western forests are doubly destructive. They not only kill the trees now growing on the site, but also can remain in dead roots and soils for many years, and kill any future trees that become established within the infested site. Some root disease fungi remain alive and active in infested sites for more than 50 years. The losses resulting from these diseases include the trees destroyed initially plus the loss in productivity of the site for the number of years it is infested.

Four major tree root diseases are found in the western United States: annosus root disease, armillaria root disease, black stain root disease, and *Phellinus weiri* root disease. The relative importance of each disease, however, varies from area to area. Several lesser diseases may be important in local areas or in certain periods of a stand's development.

The diagnosis of root diseases is difficult and can seldom be made only on the basis of above-ground symptoms. The above-ground symptoms—chlorosis, reduced tree growth, reduced needle length, fading crown, progressive thinning of foliage, and finally death—are the same for all root diseases. These symptoms also are similar to those caused by drought, high water table, air pollution, and bark beetle attack. The decline of the tree affected by root disease or air pollution usually extends over a period of a few to several years, whereas the other causes of decline kill the tree in 1 to 2 years. The spatial and temporal patterns of the dead and dying trees often are helpful in diagnosing root disease as the cause of a problem.

Characteristically, root diseases start in a tree or stump and spread slowly outward in all directions. This results in a slowly enlarging group of dead trees, with the oldest kills at the center and with a fringe of dying and recently killed trees around the outer edge. Thus, if one finds a pocket of dead trees that were killed all at once, one would suspect some other cause such as ground fire, high water table, or insect attack. Accurate diagnosis depends upon examination of part or all of the root crown and major buttress roots. This portion of the tree provides the most helpful signs and symptoms of each root disease, such as sapwood stain and decay, mycelial fans, rhizomorphs, resinosis, and fruiting bodies. It is best to choose a recently killed tree for examination of these below-ground signs. Frequently, these signs are destroyed after a year or two by secondary invaders—both insects and fungi.

DESCRIPTIVE KEY

A^1 Black to chocolate-brown stain or streaks of stain in the sapwood of the roots, or root crown, or lower bole or all of them .... *Leptographium wageneri*

A^2 No black stain; stain if present is blue, blue-gray, or gray .... B

B^1 Large white mycelial fans between bark and wood of roots and root crown. Shoestring-like strands (rhizomorphs) sometimes present on roots or under the bark or both. Associated decay is a white to yellowish stringy rot sometimes with fine black zone lines. .... *Armillaria ostoyae*

B^2 White mycelial fans and rhizomorphs absent C

C^1 Bark of roots and root crown separates easily from wood. Small white flecks of mycelium are on inner side of bark—numerous brown resin canals are noted on wood surface. Small white amorphous fruiting bodies or buttonlike fruiting body initials may be present on roots or root crown below soil surface, or shelf-like cream to light-orange-colored fruiting bodies inside hollow stumps. Associated decay is white to cream colored, soft and spongy. .... *Heterobasidion annosum*

C^2 Roots and lower bole are decayed, leaving a yellow-to-buff laminated rot with dark brown mycelial felts often between sheets of decayed wood and in shrinkage cracks. Fruiting bodies on roots are inconspicuous, crustlike, covered with many small pores, buff with white margin when young, turning dark brown with age. .... *Phellinus weiri* complex

Annosus Root Disease
Heterobasidion annosum

Hosts—*Heterobasidion annosum* infects an extensive range of hosts including most conifers, some hardwoods, and a few species of brush. To date, it has been found on nearly all native and many introduced conifers in the western United States. At least 2 host-specific forms have been identified: a p-type, which occurs mainly on pines and incense-cedar, and an s-type, which infects mostly spruce, firs, Douglas-fir, western redcedar, giant sequoia, and hemlock. Hardwoods and brush are infected by the p-type.

Distribution and damage—Worldwide in distribution, *H. annosum* is also widely distributed throughout the conifer forests of the western United States. It has been found from the dry pinyon-juniper woodland of the Southwest to the high-rainfall cedar-hemlock forests of the Pacific Northwest. This fungus is indigenous and most abundant in the true fir forests of California and hemlock forests of Oregon and Washington. It is being found with greater frequency than before in the logged pine forests of California.

In Europe and the southeastern United States, the incidence of this disease has increased directly with increased forest management so that now it has become one of the major disease problems. A similar situation has developed in the western United States where annosus root disease is now a major cause of tree mortality in certain forest types.

The way in which the host is affected and the type of resulting damage may differ between hosts and regions. In pine, the fungus spreads through the root system, first attacking the inner bark and sapwood, killing these tissues. Its penetration into the heartwood is delayed. Within 2 to 6 years after initial infection, the fungus reaches the root crown and girdles the tree. The tree dies, but the fungus remains active as a saprophytic wood-decaying organism within the roots and butt of the dead tree. Thus, in pine, *H. annosum* usually kills the host within a short period. Pines weakened by *H. annosum* are often killed by bark beetles.

In most other host species, the fungus seldom attacks the root tissues to the extent that the host is killed directly. In these hosts, the sapwood and inner bark usually are invaded in the small-to-medium-sized roots. And the fungus is initially confined to the heartwood and inner sapwood of the larger roots. Within the heartwood, the fungus spreads through the roots and root crown into the lower trunk of the host, where it causes a butt rot of the heartwood. Thus, infection in these species usually does not kill the host directly, although it may affect its growth or thriftiness. Losses from *H. annosum* in true firs are mainly the result of butt rot, increased susceptibility to insect attack, and increased windthrow.

Disease cycle—This fungus can survive for as long as 50 years as a saprophyte in the roots of large infected stumps and trees. During favorable periods, the fungus in these stumps and roots forms fruiting bodies that in turn produce numerous spores. Air currents distribute the spores to new infection sites. These sites are usually freshly cut stump surfaces of all conifer species and basal wounds of hemlock and fir. Spores landing on a fresh stump surface germinate, infect the new stump, grow down into the roots, and eventually colonize the stump and its root system.

Once established in the stump, the fungus grows into the roots of neighboring host trees wherever root contact between the infested stump and the surrounding trees exists. The p-type will infect both p-type and s-type hosts, and the s-type only the s-type hosts. From these newly established infections at the site of root contact, the fungus spreads through the roots of the new host to the root crown. The rest of this tree's root system is colonized and the fungus spreads to neighboring hosts, again through root contact. By this method, enlarging infection centers are formed.

Field identification—In pines, the pattern of dying within the stand and individual trees is often helpful in diagnosing this root disease. The presence of annosus root disease is indicated by group killing of trees over a period of years with the oldest deaths at the center and the most recently dead and dying trees on the periphery. The presence of a stump at the center near the oldest kill suggests *H. annosum* root disease. If death of individual trees has been preceded by a period of reduced radial or height growth, and if the crowns of the dying trees are thin and chlorotic, annosus root disease is again suspected.

H. annosum fruiting bodies, although not always present on dead and dying trees and associated stumps, are the best field evidence of this root disease. The fruiting bodies vary in size and form from a small button up to a bracket-type conk several inches wide, whereas in other cases they may appear as irregularly shaped, amorphous fruiting bodies (fig. 6-1). The fruiting bodies found on the root crowns of infected pines range from 0.5 inch to 2 inches (1.3 to 5.1 cm) across, with a light-brown to gray upper surface and a creamy-white lower pore surface. It is usually necessary to remove the duff from around the base of the tree to expose the fruiting bodies, which are characteristically found below the litter layer. Small, button-like fruiting bodies can often be found on the wood beneath the bark of pine stumps and on the surface of small pine roots in the soil. Conks found in the cavities of old, hollow, heart-rotted stumps are larger—sometimes up to 10 inches (25 cm) wide—and conks on true fir stumps tend to have a pale orange cast to the pore surface.

Symptoms of this disease in pine may also be found by exposing

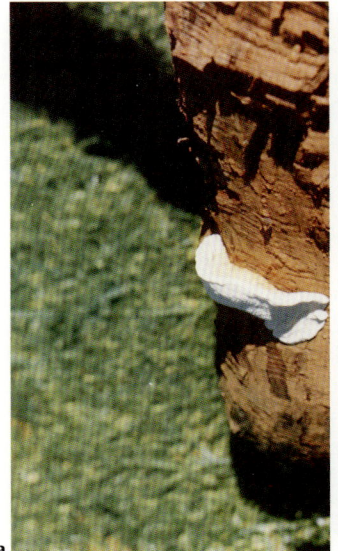
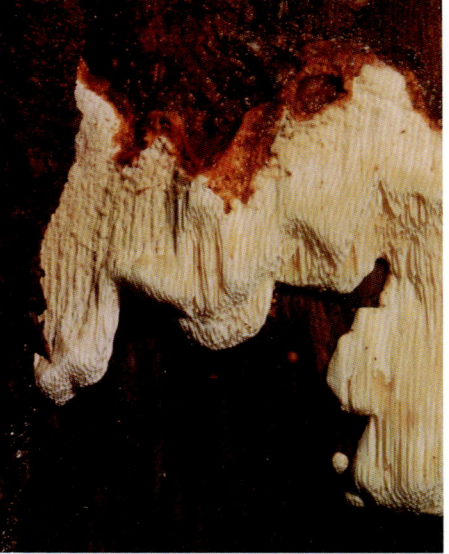

Figure 6-1—*A fruiting body of the annosus root disease fungus (*Heterobasidion annosum*) has grown on the surface of an infected pine root just below the duff (**a**). Larger amorphous-type conks are typical of those found inside stumps (**b**). Note the buff-colored upper surface and white lower surface.*

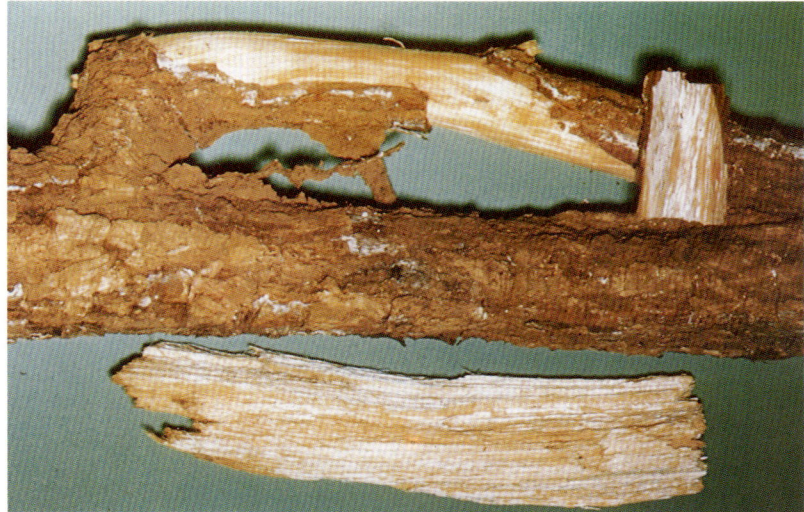

Figure 6-2—*A root infected by annosus root disease showing the tan streaking of the outer wood surface and the silver pockets of fungus growth on the inner surface of the bark. The white pocket rot characteristic of annosus root disease is shown in the piece of wood.*

the roots and root crown and examining the inner bark. Indications of
H. annosum infection in pine are (1) the bark separates easily from
the wood; (2) the separated surfaces are light brown to buff and the
surface of the wood is streaked with darker brown lines (fig. 6-2); and
(3) the surface of the inner bark has numerous small silver to white
flecks. These symptoms may be difficult to see when the roots are
wet in the spring. In addition, small white to buff mycelial pads or
outgrowths are sometimes found between the outerbark scales or on
the bark surface. Infected roots are often heavily infiltrated with resin,
and balls of resin are sometimes found in the soil next to infected
roots. In westside true fir and hemlock, mortality from this disease
alone is infrequent, and there the immediate cause of mortality
involving this disease is most often windthrow, beetle attack, or other
conditions. However, in eastside true fir, mortality caused by
H. annosum is very common, and this disease should be considered
when diagnosing the cause of true fir mortality in this region. The
best signs of this disease in true fir are the presence of fruiting bodies
in the hollow roots and trunk and the type of wood decay in the roots
and trunk. This decay is described in the chapter on rots.

Armillaria Root Disease
Armillaria ostoyae

Armillaria ostoyae is responsible for most of the root disease
known as armillaria root disease or shoestring root disease of conifers. Other species of *Armillaria* are responsible for root diseases of
hardwoods and orchard trees. Widespread throughout the tropical
and temperate regions of the world, *Armillaria* spp. have long been
recognized as the causes of major root diseases and are widespread
forest saprophytes. These two differing roles of *Armillaria* have done
much to cloud our past judgment of its importance in the forest.
Recent studies indicate *A. ostoyae* is the most common species of
Armillaria that is pathogenic to conifers in the forest environment.
Other species appear to be pathogenic to hardwoods or saprophytic.
Much still needs to be learned about the taxonomy and roles of the
species of this genus.

Hosts—Most conifers in the western United States are probably
at least moderately susceptible to *A. ostoyae*. Some are highly
susceptible.

The fungus attacks the roots and root crown of trees of all ages,
killing the cambium and inner bark and causing a decay of both
sapwood and heartwood. It is highly aggressive and damaging in
some young conifer plantations and ornamental plantings. In younger
trees, the pathogen advances rapidly through the inner bark to the
root collar, where it girdles and kills the tree. In older trees, this
advance through the inner bark proceeds much more slowly and in

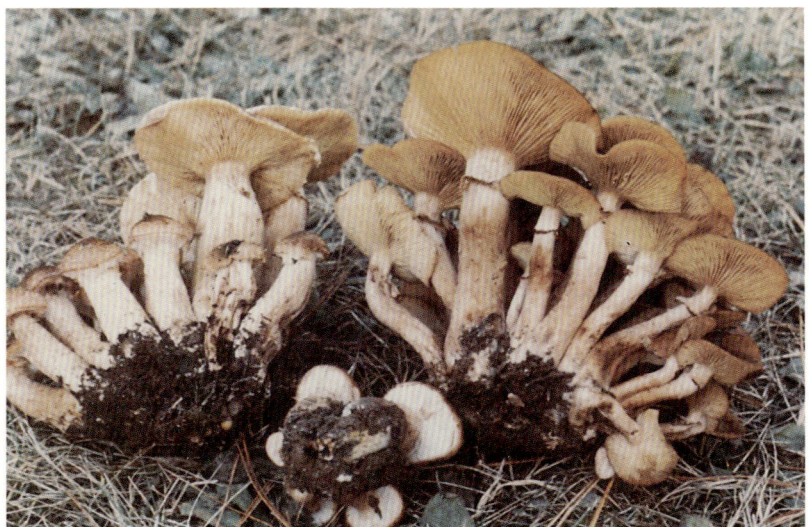

Figure 6-3—*A cluster of mushroom-like fruiting bodies of the armillaria root disease fungus* (Armillaria ostoyae). *Note the light-brown color, the annulus on the stalk, and the cap with gills.*

some species is often blocked by the host before the fungus reaches the root crown. In cases where cambial advance is checked, decay of inner wood may continue to advance and the fungus structurally weakens the roots and predisposes the tree to windthrow (see chapter 7). The virulence of this pathogen is greatly influenced by the environment, the host's vigor, and the pathogen's inoculum potential (food base).

Disease cycle—In general, this fungus lives as a decay organism in the roots, lower boles, and stumps of either dead or living trees. In some cases, however, it becomes actively parasitic on living trees. Its fruiting bodies (fig. 6-3), which are typical gill fungi (mushrooms), develop in the fall in clusters at or near the base of infected dead or dying trees and stumps. The mature fruiting bodies release many small spores that are windborne to other infection sites, such as stumps or woody debris on the forest floor. Infection of living trees by spores has not been demonstrated. *A. ostoyae* is most commonly spread to living trees by rhizomorphs or root contact (fig. 6-4). Rhizomorphs are specialized fungus structures that grow out from an established food base to colonize new sites. When these rhizomorphs, growing through the upper soil and litter layers, contact the root or root crown of a new host, they penetrate through the bark and attempt to establish an infection. The disease also spreads when the roots of an uninfected tree come in contact with an old infected root or stump and the pathogen grows into the new host root.

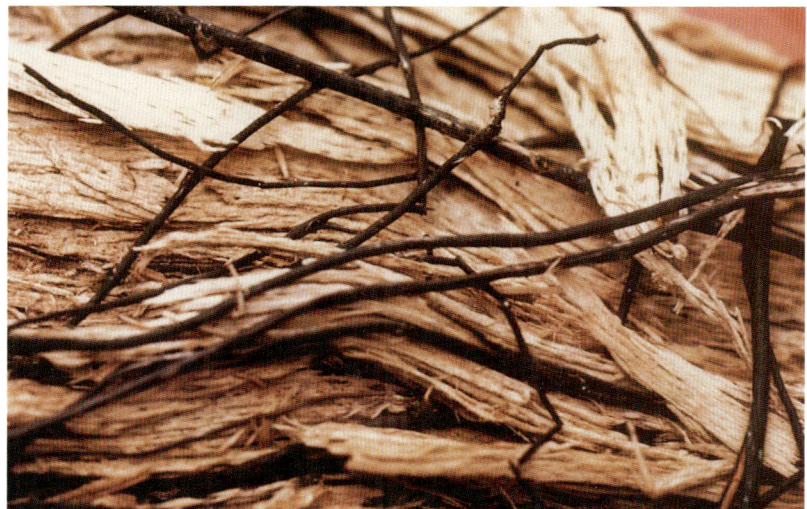
Figure 6-4—*A closeup of the rhizomorphs of armillaria root disease typically found on or under the bark of infected roots and root crowns.*

Field identification—Occasionally, the fungus can be identified in the field by its fruiting bodies (fig. 6-3), which develop in groups around the bases of infected trees in fall. These fruiting bodies are light-brown to honey-colored mushrooms with a central stalk 3 to 10 inches (8 to 25 cm) long. A ring or annulus is usually found around the stalk. The cap, 2 to 5 inches (5 to 13 cm) across, is honey yellow and may be dotted with dark brown scales. The gills are white to pale yellow and are attached to the stalk. The fruiting bodies are of limited diagnostic value in many areas of the western United States because of their infrequent production and their short season of appearance.

The rhizomorphs (fig. 6-4) and mycelial fans (fig. 6-5), which the fungus produces on the host, are of greater aid in diagnosis. Rhizomorphs may be produced between the bark and the wood, on bark surfaces below the soil line, and in the litter and soil around the roots and root crown. They are dark brown to black, flattened, and string-like structures with a white central core. They may resemble small rootlets, but on closer examination will be found to adhere to and penetrate directly into infected root surfaces and to branch differently than do true rootlets.

Mycelial fans (fig. 6-5) are creamy white, flat, thin, leathery sheets of fungus growth that develop in the cambial area between the bark and the wood of an infected host. The advancing margin of these sheets is fan-shaped and often veined.

Other characteristics used in identifying this disease are resinosis and type of decay. Excess resin and resin flow are frequently encoun-

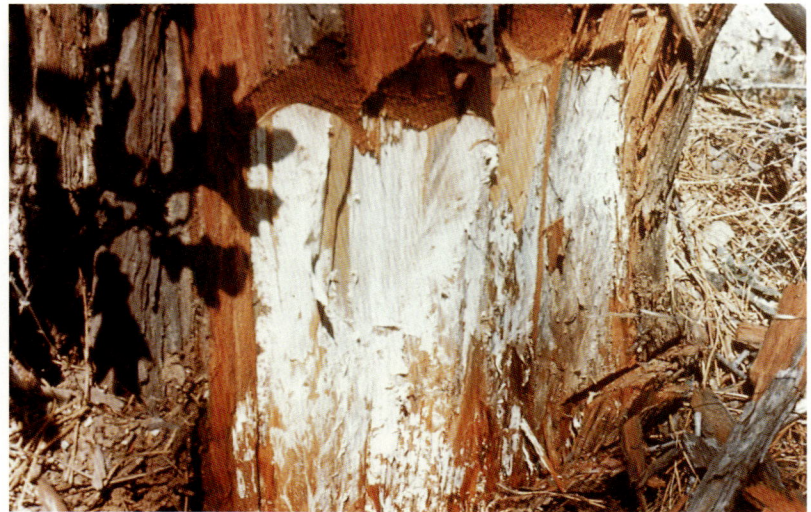

Figure 6-5—*Mycelial fans of armillaria root disease as they appear on an incense-cedar. These creamy white leathery sheets of fungus grow beneath the bark of infected roots, root crowns, and lower stems.*

tered at the root crown in the bark and surrounding soil. The wood decay caused by *A. ostoyae* is a white to yellowish stringy rot that may be accompanied by fine black zone lines.

Black Stain Root Disease
Leptographium wageneri

Hosts—This disease is caused by three different host-specific races of *Leptographium wageneri*. One race infects Douglas-fir along the Pacific Coast, another infects various hard pines (mainly ponderosa and Jeffrey pines), and the last is a pathogen of pinyon pines in California and the Southwest. The fungus occurs occasionally on western white, knobcone, lodgepole, and sugar pines and on western and mountain hemlock. Greenhouse studies and field observation show that white and red firs are resistant.

Distribution and damage—Black stain root disease is caused by the fungus *L. wageneri*. The disease not only causes great losses in commercial forests, but the damage it has done in the pinyon forests in Mesa Verde National Park and in the high-value recreational forests of southern California indicates that *L. wageneri* is a serious pest. It is widely distributed on substantial acreages in western Oregon, where it affects 10- to 30-year-old Douglas-fir in plantations. The disease is similar to oak wilt and Dutch elm disease—two very damaging vascular wilt diseases of eastern hardwoods. This disease is known to exist only in the western United States. It is widely but sparsely distributed throughout eight western States. One of the largest areas of infection is in southern California, where several thousand acres of singleleaf pinyon forests are infested, but many stands, particularly of ponderosa pines and Douglas-fir, are also severely infested with this disease. Damage by this disease may be locally quite severe.

L. wageneri attacks trees of all ages. It infects the roots, where it spreads throughout the sapwood of the root system, root crown, and lower bole. This infection of the root system causes a visible decline in tree vigor. Terminal growth is reduced, needles become shorter and chlorotic, the number of needles produced and retained is reduced, and finally the host dies. Trees weakened by this disease are predisposed to bark beetle attack. The fungus does not decay the root wood.

Disease cycle—There are two distinct phases of the spread of this disease—local spread and long distance spread. Local spread—within an existing infection center—occurs through root contacts. Infection occurs at the site of root contact between an infected and healthy root. Once established in the root, the fungus colonizes the distal portion of the root and grows toward the root crown. From the root crown, it colonizes the remaining roots. Long distance spread involves the establishment of new infection centers away from existing ones. How this occurs is not known, but insect transmission is likely. New infection centers often are associated with site disturbances and often are found concentrated along roads.

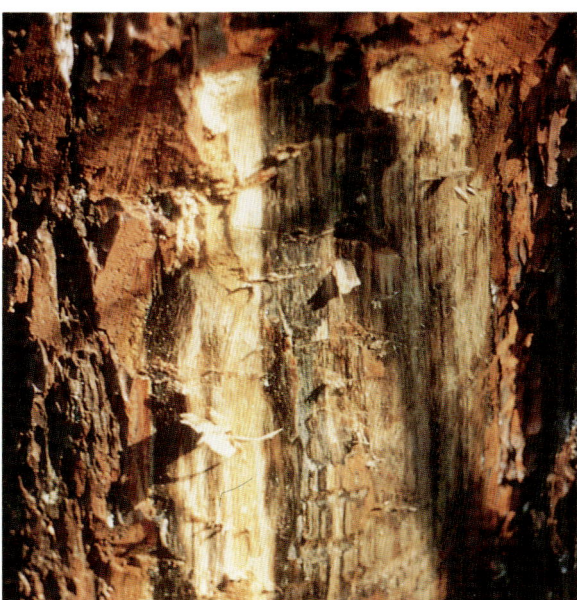

Figure 6-6—*The black to dark brown stain of black stain root disease, caused by* Leptographium wagenerii, *as it appears in the sapwood of the root crown of a western white pine.*

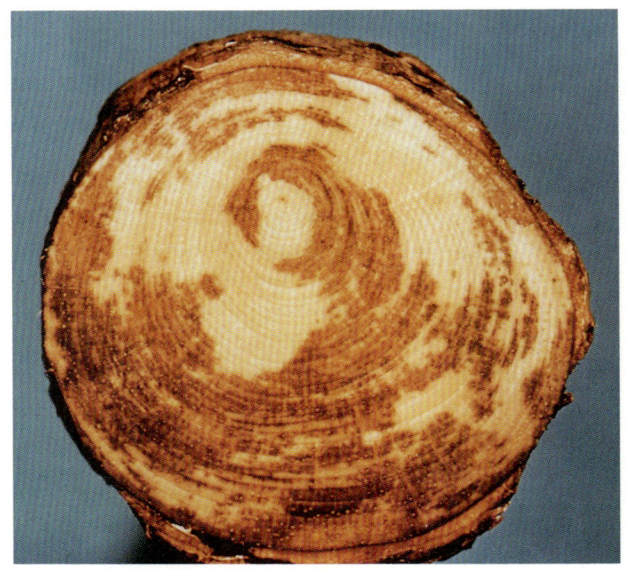

Figure 6-7—
A cross-section of a pinyon root infected with black stain root disease showing how stain tends to occur in arcs that follow the growth rings.

Field identification—This disease is relatively easy to identify in the field. It produces a distinctive sapwood stain in the roots, root crown, and sometimes the lower bole (fig. 6-6). The stained sapwood is black to dark chocolate-brown, and often is infiltrated with resin. In cross section, the stain tends to occur in arcs that follow annual rings (fig. 6-7) rather than in the wedge-shaped patterns characteristic of other sapwood stains. Blue stain, which is sometimes confused with black stain, has a wedge-shaped pattern and a bluish-gray cast.

Phellinus Weiri Root Rot
Phellinus weiri complex

Hosts—Recent research has shown that there are two basic forms of *Phellinus weiri*: one that causes a root and butt rot of western redcedar and another that causes a root disease of Douglas-fir. Douglas-fir, grand fir, white fir, and western hemlock are the most common and susceptible hosts of the Douglas-fir form, but it can infect most all conifers to some degree. The taxonomy of this complex is still being sorted out, but currently there appears to be a cedar form and a Douglas-fir form that differ in host range, kind of damage caused, cultural characteristics, sporophore longevity (perennial in cedar type and annual in Douglas-fir type) and basidiospore germination.

Distribution and damage—The range of this root disease caused by the Douglas-fir form extends from southwestern Canada to the forests of northwestern California. This form of *P. weiri* causes both a necrosis of the inner bark of the roots and the root crown and a wood decay of the roots and the lower bole, resulting in growth loss and eventually death of the infected tree. Windthrow of infected living trees caused by excess root decay is also common. This is the most damaging disease of Douglas-fir in the Pacific Northwest. It is responsible for an estimated annual loss of several million cubic feet of timber. Available evidence suggests that root disease centers probably contribute materially to maintaining populations of Douglas-fir bark beetles between outbreak years.

Disease cycle—The Douglas-fir form of *P. weiri* is a native inhabitant of many forest stands in the Pacific Northwest. Initial infection of the current stand of trees starts when their roots contact *P. weiri*-infested stumps and roots of the previous stand. The fungus spreads to the surfaces of new roots and penetrates directly through the bark to the living tissues. Once in the root, the fungus may develop in the heartwood or sapwood. Spread within a stand occurs through root contacts between infected and healthy trees. The fungus does not grow through the soil for any distance. The fungus forms fruiting bodies, which produce basidiospores, but their role is unknown. No asexual spores are formed.

Field identification—Above ground symptoms of *P. weiri* infection are chlorosis, reduction in growth, gradual thinning of the crown, and frequently a crop of distress cones. Live trees with advanced root-decay are frequently windthrown.

Incipient decay in the roots and lower bole appears as a red-brown stain, frequently in the outer heartwood. As decay proceeds, the wood softens, small pits appear, and the annual rings separate to form the typical yellow laminated rot. Brown mycelium often can be found between the sheets of decayed wood.

Fruiting bodies, which are infrequent, are found on upturned roots and on the underside of decayed logs (fig. 6-8). They appear as light buff-colored crusts with a white margin. The exposed surface of the fruiting body is covered with many small, uniform-sized, regularly shaped pores. As they age, these fruiting bodies turn dark brown.

Minor Root Diseases

Phaeolus schweinitzii, the velvet top fungus, commonly causes a root and butt rot of conifers. Infection of young plantation conifers has occasionally resulted in rather high mortality. The decay of the roots of older trees by this fungus often predisposes the host to windthrow. See chapter 7 for a description of the velvet top fungus and the decay it causes.

Phytophthora cinnamomi causes a root disease of many tree species, including conifers. *P. cinnamomi* is limited by environmental factors; it requires soils that are warm and moist—two conditions that do not occur simultaneously in most forest lands of western

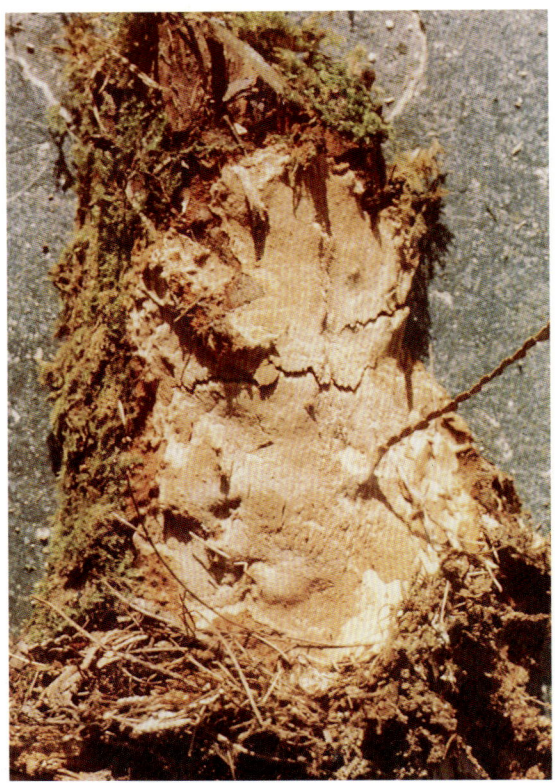

Figure 6-8—*The fruiting bodies of laminated root rot caused by* Phellinus weiri *are uncommon, but when found often appear as a "crust" with a buff-colored pore surface.*

United States. Because of these limitations, *P. cinnamomi* is usually found in the irrigated warmer soils of the Sierra Nevada foothills and southern California. Forest nurseries, Christmas tree farms, parks, and other sites with summer irrigation are the areas in which *P. cinnamomi* is most often found.

Phytophthora lateralis causes a very destructive root disease of Port-Orford-cedar in southwestern Oregon and northwestern California. This disease attacks and kills the fine roots of the host and grows up through the root system to the root crown, where it girdles the tree and causes a brown stain of the sapwood. This disease is spread long distances by humans moving infected trees or infested soil, or both, into new areas. The fungus attacks and kills the cedar in these new areas. Once established in an area, the fungus produces motile water-borne spores that can move down water courses and spread the disease to cedar further downstream. Spread of this disease by humans can be reduced by not allowing soil to be moved from infested areas into non-infested areas on road-building and logging equipment and other vehicles.

Macrophomina phaseolina, which is responsible for charcoal root disease of tree seedlings in forest nurseries, is occasionally found causing a root disease of older planted trees. It is limited to very warm sites and is most often detected during periods of moisture stress. The disease can be identified by the presence of numerous small, spherical, black, fungus bodies (microsclerotia) in the inner bark and on the xylem surface of infected roots.

SELECTED REFERENCES

Bega, R.V.; Smith, R.S., Jr. 1966. Distribution of *Fomes annosus* in the natural forests of California. Plant Disease Reporter 50:832–836.

Boyce, J.S. 1948. Root diseases. In: Forest pathology. New York: McGraw-Hill: 99–113.

Childs, T.W. 1963. *Poria weirii* root rot. Phytopathology 53:1124–1127.

Driver, C.H.; Ginns, J.H., Jr. 1968. Practical control of *Fomes annosus* in intensive forest management. Contrib. 5. Seattle: University of Washington College of Forest Resources. 8 p.

Harrington, T.C.; Cobb, F.W., Jr. 1988. Leptographium root diseases on conifers. St. Paul, MN: APS Press. 149 p.

Hodges, C.S. 1969. Modes of infection and spread of *Fomes annosus*. Annual Review Phytopathology 7:257–266.

Hodges, C.S.; Jorgensen, E. 1967. *Fomes annosus* root rot. In: Davidson, A.G.; Prentice, R.M., eds. Important forest insects and diseases of mutual concern to Canada, the United States, and Mexico. Publ. 1180. Ottawa, Canada: Department of Forestry and Rural Development.

Larsen, M.J.; Lombard, F.F. 1989. Taxonomy and nomenclature of *Phellinus weiri* in North America. In: Morrison, D.J., ed. Proceedings 7th international conference on root and butt rots; IUFRO Working Party: 1988, August 9–16, Victoria, BC; Pacific Forestry Centre. Victoria, BC: Forestry Canada. 573–578.

Otrosina, W.J.; Scharpf, R.F., tech. coords. 1989. Research and management of annosus root disease (*Heterobasidion annosum*) in western North America. Gen. Tech. Rep. PSW-116. Berkeley, CA: U.S. Department of Agriculture, Forest Service, Pacific Southwest Forest and Range Experiment Station, 177 p.

Peace, T.R. 1962. Pathology of trees and shrubs. Oxford: Clarendon Press. 753 p.

Raabe, R.D. 1962. Host list of the root rot fungus *Armillaria mellea*. Hilgardia 33:25–88.

Shaw, C.G., III; Kile, G.A. 1991. Armillaria Root Disease. Agric. Handbook 691, Washington, DC: U.S. Department of Agriculture. 233 p.

Smith, R.S., Jr. 1967. *Verticicladiella* root disease of pines. Phytopathology 57:935–938.

Wagener, W. W.; Cave, M.S. 1946. Pine killing by the root fungus, *Fomes annosus* in California. Journal Forestry 44:47–54.

Wagener, W.W.; Mielke, J.L. 1961. A staining fungus root disease of ponderosa, Jeffrey, and pinyon pines. Plant Disease Reporter 45:831–835.

Wallis, G.W.; Reynolds, G. 1965. The initiation and spread of *Poria weirii* root rot of Douglas-fir. Canadian Journal Botany 43:1–9.

Williams, R.E.; Shaw, C.G. III; Wargo, P.M.; Sites, W.H. 1986. Armillaria root disease. For. Pest Leafl. 78. Washington, DC: U.S. Department of Agriculture.

CHAPTER 7   Heart Rots

Robert F. Scharpf and Donald Goheen
Research Scientist Emeritus, formerly Principal Plant Pathologist and Project Leader, Disease Research, Pacific Southwest Research Station, Forest Service, U.S. Department of Agriculture, Albany, CA.
Plant Pathologist, Forest Pest Management, Pacific Northwest Region, Forest Service, U.S. Department of Agriculture, Portland, OR.

INTRODUCTION

Heart rots are caused by fungi that attack and rot (decay) the nonliving heartwood in the central core of a tree. The living outer cylinder of wood, commonly called sapwood, is usually free of attack.

About a dozen different fungi are considered major heart rot organisms of conifers along the Pacific Coast. A few of these fungi are host-specific—that is, they attack only one tree species. Others rot heartwood of nearly every major conifer and even some hardwoods. Many heart rot organisms decay only the heartwood of living trees, whereas some also decay heartwood and sapwood of dead trees, deteriorate wood in use, and decompose roots, slash, and organic matter in the soil. Heart rots are among the most serious forest disease problems in western North America. Collectively, they are responsible for the loss of millions of board feet of timber each year. Old-growth stands are particularly prone to attack by heart rot fungi, but even second-growth stands suffer heavy losses in certain instances. Rots not only render timber unmerchantable, but reduce the quality of the wood that is used. Rot fungi also predispose trees to windthrow and breakage, thus causing additional loss of timber and hazards in recreational and high-use areas.

As a rule, heart rot fungi do not penetrate sound trees, but require an opening into the heartwood through which to invade. Any opening into the heartwood or exposure of dead sapwood next to heartwood is a potential site for heart rot fungi to become established. Wounds caused by fire or human activities are common points of entry by these fungi. The elimination of all wounds is not possible. Animals, particularly rodents, birds, and insects, wound trees. Weather, such as lightning, wind, snow, ice, and excessive heat and cold, wounds trees, providing entrance courts for heart rot fungi. But these types of wounds are usually considered less important than those caused by human activity and by fire.

Certain natural openings in trees also provide a means of entrance for heart rot organisms—among these are branch stubs, open knots, and dead branches. A few heart rot fungi penetrate living branches. Some heart rot fungi enter the tree through injured roots or through basal fire scars. These are often called **butt rots**. Other fungi such as *Heterobasidion annosum* and *Phaeolus schweinitzii* are root parasites as well as heart rot fungi and kill roots before invading the heartwood. These are commonly referred to as **root diseases**.

Several systems have been devised to classify the heart rots conveniently. But, for the most part, only three of these are useful for field identification. One system is based on the type of rot produced; the second, on the characteristics of the fungus fruiting body; and the third, on the location of the rot within the tree.

The first system recognizes two general types of rots: (1) the **brown rots** and (2) the **white rots**. Brown rots develop as a result of the selective utilization of carbohydrates (primarily cellulose) by the fungus, leaving behind the brownish lignin component of wood. Brown rotted wood usually is dry and fragile and tends to crumble readily or break into cubes of various sizes. Most brown rots form a solid column of rot, but some appear in pockets, such as those caused by *Oligoporus amarus* and *O. sequoiae*. A few brown rot fungi produce a stringy, brown rot that in some cases is similar to that produced by certain white rot fungi.

The white rots are produced by fungi that attack both the carbohydrate and lignin components of wood. They may be further divided into (1) **pocket rots**, (2) **white stringy rots**, (3) **yellow stringy rots**, and (4) **others**, depending on their appearance and texture.

For some species, the appearance of the rot is a distinctive characteristic, as for example, the pocket rot caused by *O. amarus*. In other cases, the type of rot produced by a given species is not distinctive and only suggests the fungus responsible.

The second classification system used to identify heart rot fungi in the field is based on the characteristics of the fruiting body, more commonly known as a **conk** or **sporophore**. These spore-producing bodies vary in form from fleshy, typically mushroom-shaped structures to woody **brackets** found on trees. Color, texture, and the nature of the spore-producing surface are other examples of characteristics used to identify the fruiting bodies of these heart rot fungi. It is usually possible to identify the heart rot species by observing the characteristics of the fruiting body and the type and location of decay associated with it.

The third classification system is based on the location of the rot in trees. Some fungi cause primarily root and butt rots; others cause trunk rot; and others cause root, butt, and trunk rots. This system is a convenient method of classifying the heart rot fungi on the basis of their general location within the tree and is used with other systems to help determine which rot fungi are involved.

Problems sometimes arise when trying to identify a specific heart rot fungus. Often heart rots occur without the presence of fruiting bodies. And, more than one type of heart rot can be present in a tree. The early stage of decay, known as **incipient rot**, is not easily recognized and may be confused with **wetwood**, stain, or other heartwood discoloration. Recent studies have shown that for many heart rot conditions in trees, a succession or community of wood-invading organisms is necessary. Bacteria as well as wood-rotting fungi and other fungi that do not decay wood may be involved. Therefore, in trying to determine the type of decay and the organism(s) responsible for the rot, use the characteristics of both the rot and the fruiting body in deciding on the rot organisms involved. More than one rot organism may be associated with a particular heart rot condition. Use of all the features available in examining trees for heart rot will increase the observers' chances for correct field identification.

SOME OF THE IMPORTANT HEART ROTS OF CONIFERS OF THE PACIFIC COAST

Trunk rots
1. Brown trunk rot—*Fomitopsis officinalis*
2. Brown crumbly rot—*Fomitopsis pinicola*
3. White mottled rot—*Ganoderma applanatum*
4. Red ring rot—*Phellinus pini*
5. Juniper pocket rot—*Pyrofomes demidoffii*
6. Brown top rot—*Fomitopis cajanderi*
7. Brown stringy rot—*Echinodontium tinctorium*
8. Red rot—*Dichomitus squalens*
9. Pocket dry rot—*Oligoporus amarus*
10. Pouch fungus—*Cryptoporus volvatus*
11. Oyster mushroom—*Pleurotus ostreatus*

Root and butt rots
1. Fomes root and butt rot—*Heterobasidion annosum*
2. Brown cubical rot—*Oligoporus balsameus*
3. Red-brown butt rot—*Phaeolus schweinitzii*
4. Brown cubical rot—*Laetiporus sulphureus*
5. Red root and butt rot—*Inonotus tomentosus*
6. Laminated root rot—*Phellinus weirii*
7. Shoestring root rot—*Armillaria ostoyae*
8. Lacquer fungus—*Ganoderma oregonense*
9. Yellow root rot—*Perenniporia subacida*

Rots of butt or trunk or both
1. Redwood cubical rot—*Oligoporus sequoiae*
2. White ring rot—*Ceriporiopsis rivulosa*

3. Mottled rot—*Pholiota adiposa*
4. Yellow pitted rot—*Hericium abietis*
5. Scaly cap fungus—*Lentinus lepideus*

DESCRIPTIVE KEY

A^1	On incense-cedar, juniper, or redwood	B
B^1	On incense-cedar	C
C^1	A brown pocket dry rot (pocket dry rot)	*Oligoporus amarus*
C^2	A white stringy root or butt rot (annosus root and butt rot)	*Heterobasidion annosum*
B^2	On juniper (juniper pocket rot)	*Pyrofomes demidoffii*
B^3	On coast redwood	D
D^1	Advanced decay, a brown pocket rot (brown cubical rot)	*Oligoporus sequoiae*
D^2	Advanced decay, a white ring rot (white ring rot)	*Ceriporiopsis rivulosa*
A^2	On other conifer hosts	E
E^1	Advanced decay brown, cubically cracked (brown rot)	F
F^1	Fruiting body large, white, mushroom-shaped; upper surface scaly, lower surface with gills (scaly cap fungus)	*Lentinus lepideus*
F^2	Fruiting body not as above; lower surface with pores, not gills	G
G^1	Fruiting bodies on the soil or on the base of the tree	H
H^1	Fruiting body brown to greenish and velvet-like in texture when fresh; often clustered. Typically a root and butt rot (red-brown butt rot)	*Phaeolus schweinitzii*
H^2	Large, fleshy annual, bracket-type, fruiting bodies; bright sulfur yellow when fresh, chalky white when old (brown cubical rot)	*Laetiporus sulphureus*
G^2	Fruiting bodies occurring anywhere on the tree	J
J^1	Perennial woody, chalky-white fruiting bodies, very bitter to taste (brown trunk rot)	*Fomitopsis officinalis*
J^2	Large rubbery to woody bracket-type fruiting bodies; dark upper surface, reddish margin, buff to cream colored pore surface (brown crumbly rot)	*Fomitopsis pinicola*
E^2	Advanced decay not distinctly brown and cubically cracked; usually white to light brown, in pockets, spongy or stringy (white rots)	K
K^1	Advanced decay as small white pockets in the heartwood (occasionally sapwood of trees)	L
L^1	Pockets white, fibrous	M

M¹ Fruiting bodies on tree trunk often clustered, light to dark brown, bracket-type, woody, with pores on lower surface (red ring rot) .... *Phellinus pini*
M² Fruiting bodies produced at the base of trees or on soil, brown to light tan; hairy zonate upper surface. Root and butt rot (red root and butt rot) .... *Inonotus tomentosus*
L² Pockets of rot empty; fruiting bodies creamy-white coral-like (yellow pitted rot) .... *Hericium abietis*
K² Advanced decay white to yellowish, stringy or spongy, pockets not conspicuous .... N
N¹ Rot not confined to root and butt of tree. Rot white, spongy with many black zone lines. Fruiting body hard, woody, up to 2 feet (0.6 m) in width. Upper surface smooth, gray to black; lower surface cream colored, turning brown when bruised .... *Ganoderma applanatum*
N² Rot confined to roots and butt of tree .... O
O¹ Fine, black zone lines present in rotted wood. White mycelial fans often present between bark and wood and black rhizomorphs often associated with the rot. Fruiting bodies mushroom-shaped with gills on the lower surface, honey-colored and occurring in clusters from the decayed wood or soil at the base of the tree (shoestring root rot) .... *Armillaria ostoyae*
O² Rot usually always associated with roots and butt of the tree. No zone lines or rhizomorphs present. Fruiting bodies irregular in shape and varying in size from small button-shaped structures to large conspicuous brackets (fomes root and butt rot) .... *Heterobasidion annosum*
O³ Rot confined to roots and butt of tree. Advanced decay, yellow-white, spongy. Decayed wood may separate along annual rings much like *Phellinus weirii*. Fruiting bodies crust-like, up to 0.5 inch (1.3 cm) thick, 2-3 feet (0.6 to 0.9 m) long, white when fresh, creamy to yellow-orange when older. Often found on underside of down logs .... *Perenniporia subacida*
K³ Advanced decay, yellow to yellowish-brown .... P
P¹ Wood in advanced decay separating into distinct laminations along growth rings. Root and butt rot (laminated root and butt rot) .... *Phellinus weirii*
P² Distinct separation of wood along growth rings not obvious .... Q
Q¹ Yellow to yellow-brown stringy rot in heartwood, tree trunk usually hollow. Fruiting bodies large, black, bracket-type, woody with a toothed undersurface and a brick-red interior (brown stringy rot) .... *Echinodontium tinctorium*

Q² Decayed heartwood having a dark, streaked or mottled appearance. No rhizomorphs. Yellowish brown mycelial strands present in the advanced decay. Fruiting bodies mushroom-shaped, yellow, with gills on lower surface and often arising in clusters from the decayed wood or base of the tree (mottled rot) .... *Pholiota adiposa*

BROWN ROTS

Quinine Fungus
Brown Trunk Rot
Fomitopsis officinalis (Fomes officinalis)

Hosts—Douglas-fir, pines, western larch, spruce, and hemlock are common hosts. The fungus seldom occurs on true firs.

Distribution and damage—This fungus is known in both Europe and North America. In western North America, it has traditionally been considered an important trunk rot of old-growth conifers. It is found most commonly on Douglas-fir and larch but also attacks pines and some other species. The incidence of this organism in second-growth forests is not well known but appears to be low. It is believed that wounds, broken tops, and branch stubs are common entrance points for the fungus. It may also occasionally enter fire scars.

Field identification—

Rot—The rot caused by this fungus is almost indistinguishable from the cubical brown rot caused by *Laetiporus sulphureus*. Unlike the sulfur fungus, the brown trunk rot only occasionally occurs in the butt and is found mainly in the trunk and upper bole of the tree, where it is often very extensive. Another characteristic that distinguishes *F. officinalis* from *L. sulphureus* is the bitter taste of fresh mycelial felts present in the decayed wood. Thus, it has been called quinine fungus.

Fruiting body—Fruiting bodies do not commonly occur on trees attacked by the fungus. When present, they are pendant, woody, perennial, often hoof-shaped structures with a chalky surface. They may range in size from several inches to more than 2 feet (0.6 m) long (fig. 7-1). Their presence indicates extensive decay. The fruiting bodies are white and leathery when young, but chalky and crumbly when old. Like the mycelial felts, they also have a bitter taste.

Red Belt Fungus/Brown Crumbly Rot
Fomitopsis pinicola (Fomes pinicola)

Hosts—Most western conifers including pines, true firs, Douglas-fir, western hemlock, western larch, spruce, and western redcedar are hosts for this fungus.

Distribution and damage—This fungus is one of the most common wood rot organisms in coniferous forests of western North

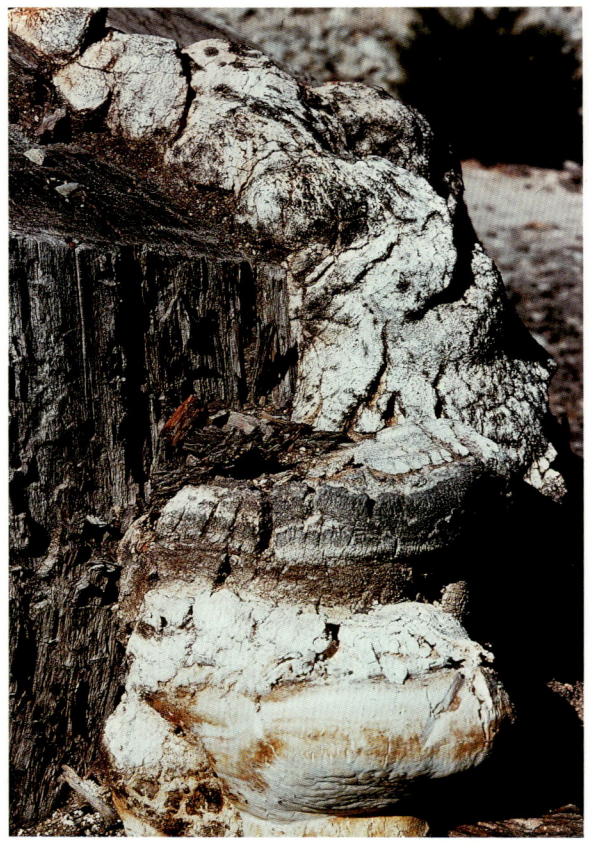

Figure 7-1—*Woody, perennial fruiting body of the quinine fungus (*Fomitopsis officinalis*) growing from the base of a Douglas-fir stump.*

America. Although it is mainly a decomposer of dead and down timber, it has also been known to cause heart rot in living trees, particularly in Alaska. The mode of entrance for this fungus is mainly through wounds and broken or dead tops. Decay in living true firs from the red belt fungus has also been found to be associated with the large open bole swellings caused by dwarf mistletoe.

Field identification—

Rot—The rot caused by this fungus is somewhat lighter in color than that caused by some of the other crumbly brown rots. Rot develops in both sapwood and heartwood. It may vary in color from a yellow brown to slightly reddish. Cubical cracking is common (fig. 7-2), and the shrinkage cracks are usually filled with white fungus felts.

Fruiting body—Fruiting bodies are commonly found associated with this rot (fig. 7-3). They are leathery to woody, perennial bracket-type structures that, when young, appear as a round white fungus

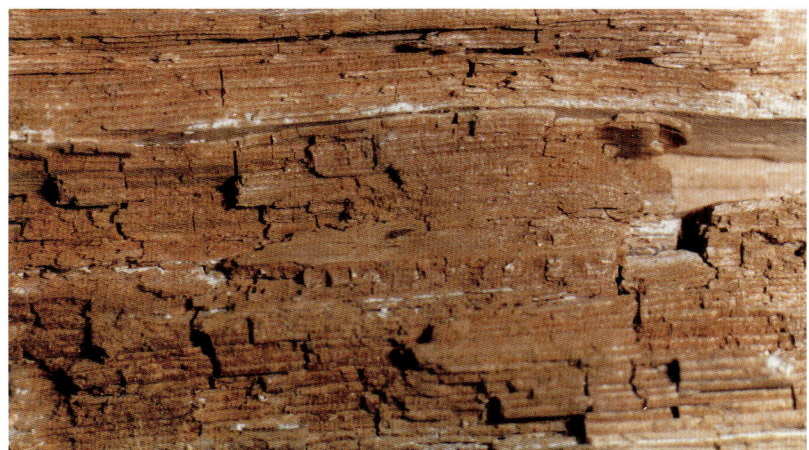

Figure 7-2—*Characteristic advanced brown rot caused by the red belt fungus* (Fomitopsis pinicola).

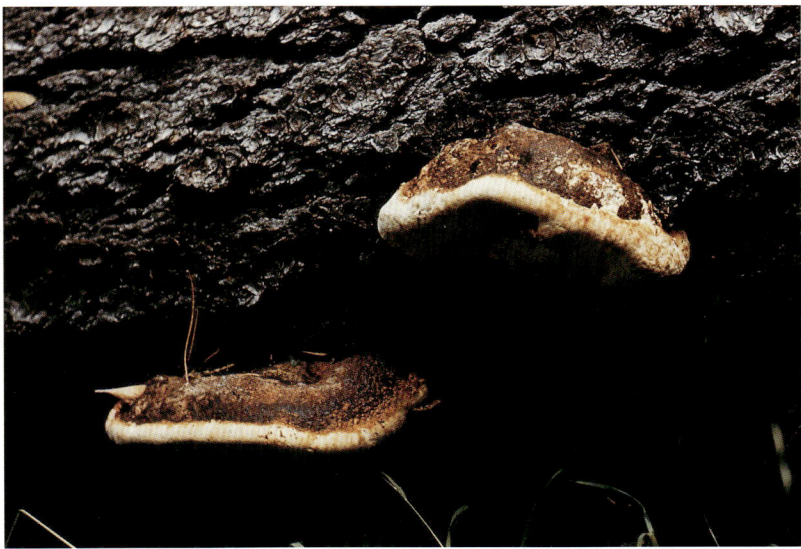

Figure 7-3—*Commonly observed fruiting body of the red belt fungus growing on a white fir log.*

mass. As they develop, the upper surface turns dark gray to black, while the fresh lower pore surface remains white to creamy in color. A conspicuous reddish margin develops between the two surfaces; thus, the name **red belt fungus**. Fruiting bodies of this organism are among the most common ones seen on dead and fallen coniferous trees. They generally range from about 4 to 18 inches (10 to 46 cm) across.

Scaly Cap Fungus
Lentinus lepideus

Hosts—Common hosts include pine, western redcedar, incense-cedar, hemlock, true fir, and Douglas-fir.

Distribution and damage—This fungus is of worldwide distribution and in the western United States is a heart rot organism. It also decays dead and down wood. As a heart-rot organism, it does not appear to be limited to any particular part of the tree. It has been observed rotting roots as well as heartwood in the upper portion of the bole. It is common on pines in the high elevations and on the eastern slope of the Sierra Nevada and in the Cascades.

Field identification—

Rot—Incipient decay appears as a yellowish stain. Advanced decay is dark brown, cubically cracked, almost black where exposed. Thin, white mycelial fans are in shrinkage cracks. Rotten wood is said to have an anise or turpentine odor.

Fruiting body—Of all the important brown heart rots of the Pacific Coast, this is the only one caused by a typical, mushroom-type fungus (fig. 7-4). The fruiting bodies are often large and range from 2 to 12 inches (5 to 30 cm) in diameter, are borne on a stalk, are leathery, and have a white gilled lower surface. The top of the cap is composed of a whitish surface overlaid with darker tan to brown scales, thus the name *scaly cap*. The dry fruiting bodies become quite hard and brittle.

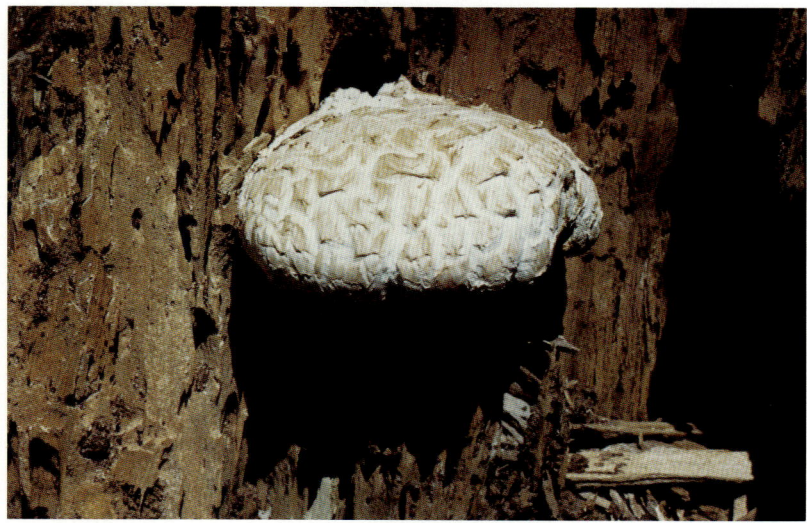

Figure 7-4—*Mushroom-like fruiting body of the scaly cap fungus (*Lentinus lepideus*).*

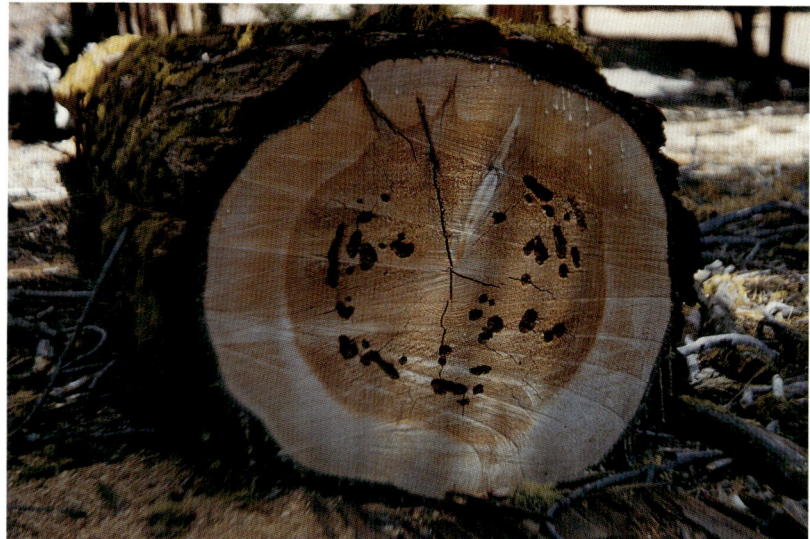

Figure 7-5—*Pocket dry rot of incense-cedar caused by* Oligoporus amarus.

Pocket Dry Rot
Oligoporus amarus (Polyporus amarus)

Hosts—Incense-cedar is the only known host.

Distribution and damage—*Oligoporus amarus* causes a common heart rot of incense-cedar throughout its natural range. More than a third of the volume, or about 5 billion board feet of the merchantable incense-cedar is culled because of rot by this fungus. Pocket dry rot is most common in trees on good growing sites and moist microsites and less common in trees on marginal sites near the eastern limit of incense-cedar. Trees less than 150 years old are relatively free of rot, whereas in trees 200 years or older, the incidence of decay increases rapidly. Fire scars, large open knots, and branch stubs are the most common entry point for the fungus.

Field identification—

Rot—*O. amarus* produces a characteristic brown pocket rot not unlike the brown cubical rot of redwood (fig. 7-5). The initial stage of the rot appears as a brownish discoloration of the heartwood. Eventually elongated pockets, usually several times longer than wide, develop. The wood within the pockets is broken down into a dry, dark brown, crumbly residue, separated by cross and longitudinal shrinkage cracks. Although pockets may coalesce with one another, the margin between rotten wood and sound wood remains sharp. The pockets never become so numerous that the entire central

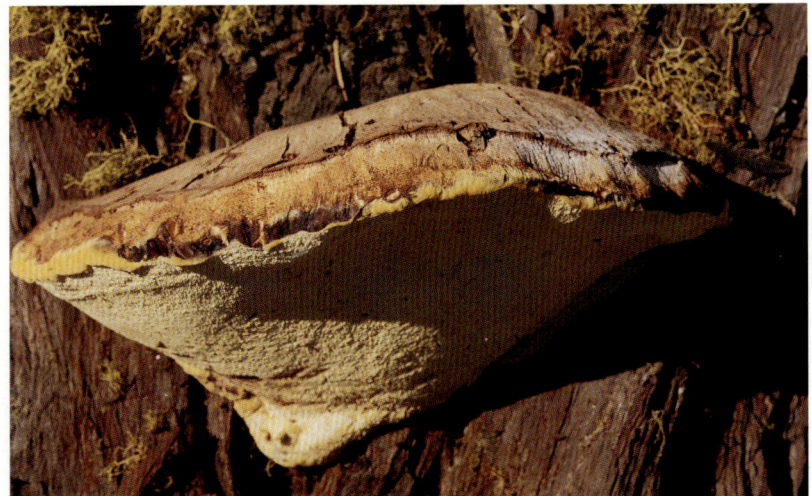

Figure 7-6—*Fruiting body of* Oligoporus amarus *on the trunk of an old-growth incense-cedar.*

cylinder of heartwood is decayed, as happens when brown cubical rot decays redwood.

Fruiting body—The fruiting bodies furnish certain evidence of extensive pocket dry rot. Usually one (rarely two) fruiting bodies are produced and then only on trees with extensive rot (fig. 7-6). When fresh they are soft, moist bracket-type structures with a yellow undersurface and tan top. They have a smooth margin and often appear somewhat hoof-shaped. Old fruiting bodies darken in color and become dry and firm. They appear annually—and only in late summer and fall. Eaten by insects, they may be destroyed in a short time. As a result, they are only occasionally seen on trees with pocket dry rot. Shot-hole cups (depressions in the bark caused by woodpeckers searching for insects at the base of an old fruiting body) are also common indicators of decayed trees.

Velvet Top Fungus
Red-Brown Butt Rot
Phaeolus schweinitzii

Hosts—Douglas-fir, pines, true firs, larch, spruce, incense-cedar, western red cedar, and rarely hemlock are known hosts.

Distribution and damage—The velvet top fungus occurs throughout the world where conifers are native or introduced. Hardwoods are seldom attacked. This fungus is most common on Douglas-fir along the Pacific Coast. The fungus generally enters trees through basal fire scars and is known mainly as a butt rot organism but is also a root parasite. Although it has been reported as a trunk rot, it almost always is confined to the root system and lower 8 to 10 feet (2.4 to 3.0 m) of the tree bole. Timber losses are not precisely known but are considered high both because the valuable butt logs are badly decayed and because infected trees are predisposed to windthrow and breakage. Infected trees often exhibit a pronounced butt swell.

Field identification—

Rot—Incipient decay from this fungus is not easy to recognize, but may appear as a yellow-green to reddish discoloration of heartwood. Advanced decay is a typical brown rot limited to the heartwood (fig. 7-7b). Rotted wood characteristically appears reddish brown and tends to form large cubes and cracks across the grain. Thin, white, resinous fungus mats may appear in the shrinkage cracks. Dry decayed wood may be easily crumbled into a fine powder.

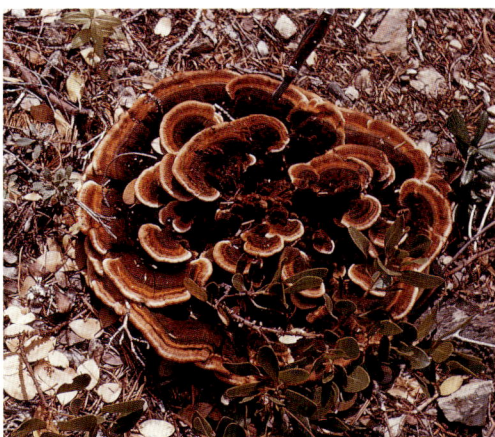

Figure 7-7—*Fruiting body of the velvet fungus* (Phaeolus schweinitzii) *on the soil at the base of an infected Douglas-fir (**a**). Red-brown butt rot of Douglas-fir caused by the velvet fungus (**b**).*

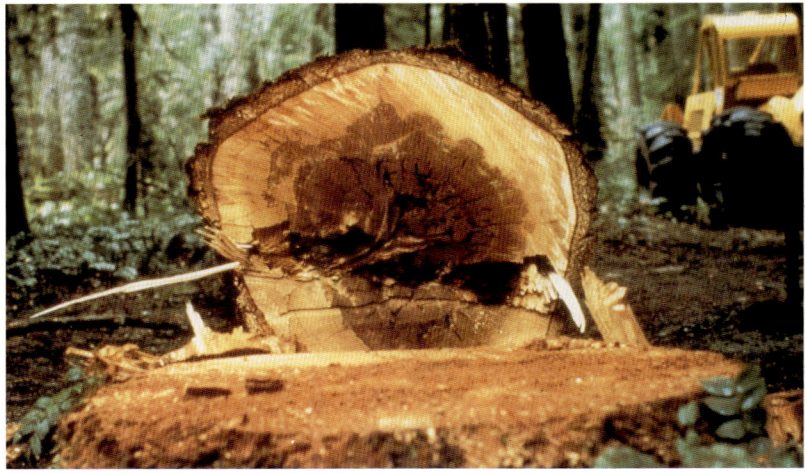

Fruiting body—The fruiting bodies of this fungus may appear either on the soil around the base of an infected tree or on the butt of the tree itself. Depending on the site of development, they may be either brackets or mushroomlike in structure. Brackets tend to form on exposed wood, whereas the stalked mushroom-type fruiting bodies usually appear on the soil (fig. 7-7a). The fruiting bodies have a soft velvety top that, when fresh, is usually reddish brown in color and encircled by a yellowish margin. Concentric lines are also present on the top surface. The lower spore-producing pore surface varies from dark green to light brown. The fruiting bodies are produced annually in summer and fall and, when old, dry up, darken, and closely resemble cow dung. Windborne spores enter and infect the host through fire scars and wounded roots. Infection can also spread from tree to tree through root contact.

Sulfur Fungus
Brown Cubical Rot
Laetiporus sulphureus (Polyporus sulphureus)

Hosts—The usual hosts of this fungus are Douglas-fir, true firs, pines, hemlock, spruce, larch, and western red cedar.

Distribution and damage—The sulfur fungus is common on hardwoods and conifers throughout much of North America. In the western United States it causes considerable rot in conifers, particularly true firs. The organism generally enters through basal fire scars and wounds on conifers and primarily causes a butt rot. Although the sulfur fungus is not considered a major slash decay organism, it is often seen on stumps, logs, and dead trees.

Field identification—

Rot—Advanced decay is similar to that caused by red-brown butt rot. Decayed wood is dark to reddish brown, cubically cracked, and is easily crumbled. Usually, white mycelial felts are present in the shrinkage cracks. These may be very thin or range up to 0.25 inch (0.6 cm) thick, a foot (0.3 m) or so wide, and several feet long.

Fruiting body—Clustered, annual, shelf-like fruiting bodies are typical of this organism (fig. 7-8). When fresh, they are soft and fleshy, with a bright yellow-orange upper surface and a bright sulfur-yellow lower pore surface. Old fruiting bodies are hard, brittle, and chalky white.

Redwood Cubical Rot
Oligoporus sequoiae (Poria sequoiae)

Hosts—Coast redwood is the only known host.

Distribution and damage—This rot is distributed throughout the natural range of redwood. As one of the two major rots in redwood, it is the most common and causes the most cull. About 10 billion board

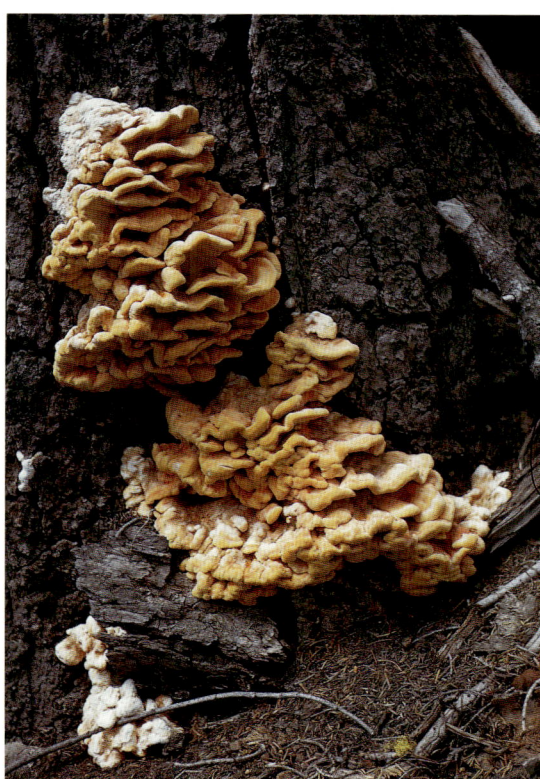

Figure 7-8—*Fresh fruiting body of the sulfur fungus (*Laetiporus sulphureus*) emerging from the stump of an old California red fir.*

feet of cull in redwood is attributed to heart rots, of which more than 75 percent is caused by *Oligoporus sequoiae*. Surveys have shown that by far the greatest amount of rot occurs in old-growth redwood, particularly in those with basal fire scars or broken tops. Second-growth redwood may suffer some loss from *O. sequoiae*, but fortunately the rot is not transferred from stumps to stump sprouts.

Field identification—

Rot—Initial stages of rot range from a dark brown stain of the inner heartwood to scattered pockets of brown charcoal-like "dry rot," which shrinks and cracks into cubes (fig. 7-9). In the advanced stages, the pockets of rot are so numerous that nearly the entire central and, to some degree, the outer cylinder of heartwood is rotted.

Fruiting body—The spore-producing structure is unlike the typical bracket or mushroom-shaped fruiting bodies produced by most of the rot fungi. Instead, the entire fruiting body develops as a thin, white mantle or crust composed of fungus strands and a spore-producing pore surface. The fruiting bodies often are no more than

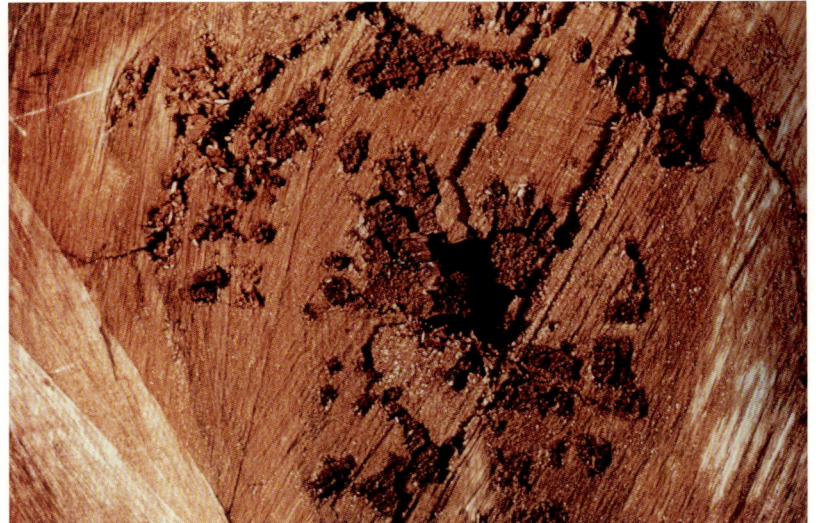

Figure 7-9—*Pockets of brown rot of redwood caused by* Oligoporus sequoiae.

2 inches (5 cm) long and 1 inch (3 cm) wide and most frequently are found in fire scars, bark crevices, and on the ends of down logs.

WHITE ROTS

Shoestring Fungus/Honey Mushroom
Shoestring Root Rot/Soft Spongy Rot
Armillaria ostoyae

Hosts—Most conifer species in western North America are hosts for this fungus.

Distribution and damage—*Armillaria ostoyae* is more commonly considered a root disease fungus than a rot organism. Therefore, details of the fungus—its distribution, occurrence, and structure of its fruiting body—are described in chapter 6.

Field identification—

Rot—Incipient decay appears as discolored water-soaked or resin-soaked wood. Advanced rot caused by the shoestring fungus is white or light yellow, soft and spongy, often stringy, marked by numerous black zone lines and confined to the roots or butt of the tree or both. Often the rot is accompanied by white mycelial fans (fig. 6-5) under the bark. Black rhizomorphs (shoestring-like fungal strands) also are usually present (fig. 6-4).

Fruiting body—For a detailed description of the fruiting body, see chapter 6 on root diseases.

Indian Paint Fungus
Brown Stringy Rot
Echinodontium tinctorium

Hosts—True firs and hemlock are the common hosts. Douglas-fir and spruce are rarely infected.

Distribution and damage—This decay fungus is distributed throughout the western United States on firs and hemlock and is considered to be the most serious heart rot organism on these tree species. In some old-growth stands, losses of 25 to 50 percent or more of the gross volume have been recorded. The Indian paint fungus may enter trees through trunk scars, dead tops, and other wounds, but most infections apparently enter through small branch stubs on suppressed trees. The Indian paint fungus remains dormant in these stubs until the tree is damaged or injured, at which time the fungus is activated to develop significant decay. As a result, the rot is most common in the mid-trunk region, but it may also extend into the butt or down from the top. Trees up to 40 to 50 years old are essentially free of brown stringy rot because only limited heartwood has developed.

Field identification—

Rot—The name **brown stringy rot** is confusing in that the Indian paint fungus attacks both lignin and cellulose components of heartwood. The fungus is, therefore, a white rot organism. The first noticeable evidence of rot is a yellowish to golden-tan discoloration of the heartwood. The invaded wood is also somewhat softer than uninvaded heartwood at this stage. Next, the heartwood turns pale reddish brown, and rust-red streaks appear along the grain. Wood with advanced rot becomes soft and stringy, and may vary from yellow brown to tan to rust red. Brown to rust-red streaks or areas are also present. Rotted wood often tends to separate along the annual rings. In the very late stages of decay, the stringy mass of rotted wood may disintegrate, leaving a hollow in the tree (fig. 7-10).

Fruiting body—The fruiting bodies of the Indian paint fungus are quite distinctive and receive their name because certain Indian tribes are believed to have ground the brick-red interior into a powder for use as a red pigment (fig. 7-11). The woody, perennial, hoof-shaped bodies range from a few inches to more than a foot in width and are quite common on infected trees. The upper surface is dull, black, and rough (fig. 7-12), whereas the undersurface is usually level but set with hard, coarse teeth or spines. This toothed surface is gray when fresh but turns black when old. Fruiting bodies develop on the bole, usually on the underside of branches or branch stubs. Heart rot often extends about 16 feet (5 m) above and below a fruiting body. Trees with one or more fruiting bodies usually have extensive decay. Punk knots are also indicators of decay by this fungus.

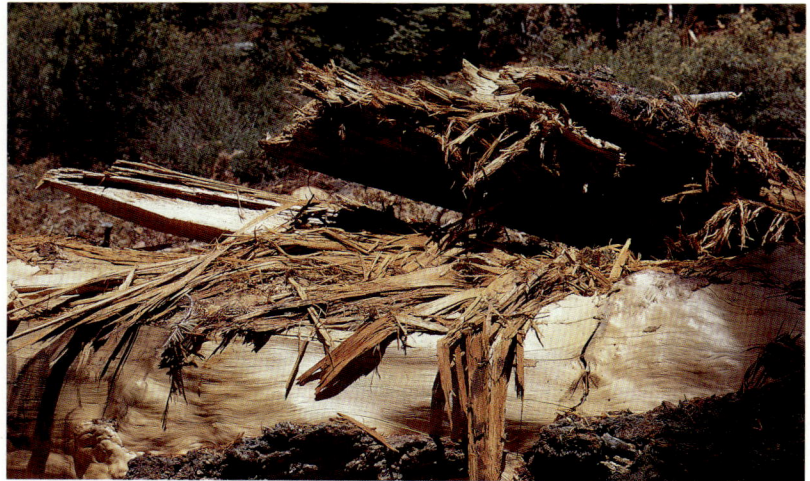

Figure 7-10—*Brown stringy rot of white fir caused by the Indian paint fungus* (Echinodontium tinctorium).

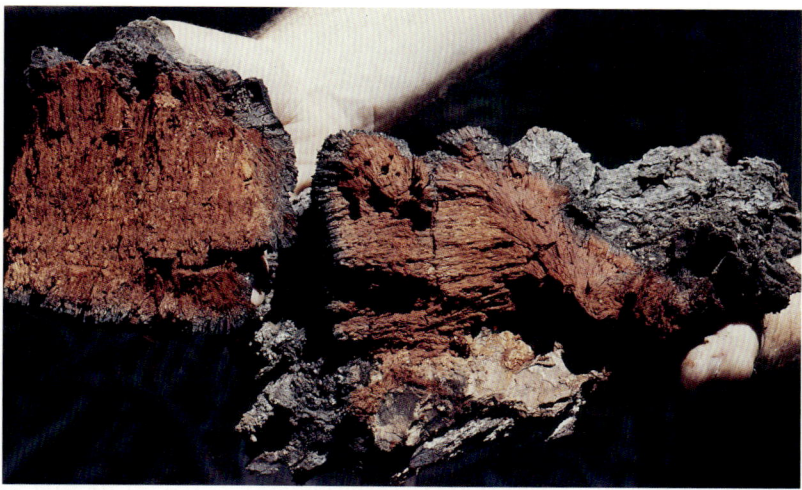

Figure 7-11—*Reddish interior of the fruiting body of the Indian paint fungus.*

Annosus Root and Butt Rot
Heterobasidion annosum (*Fomes annosus*)

Hosts—Occurs on most conifer species in the western United States.

Distribution and damage—This organism occurs throughout the coniferous forests of northern Europe, southeastern United States and western North America. Although it is primarily known as a root disease organism (see chapter 6), it also acts as an important butt and trunk rot on some species. *Heterobasidion annosum* is particularly

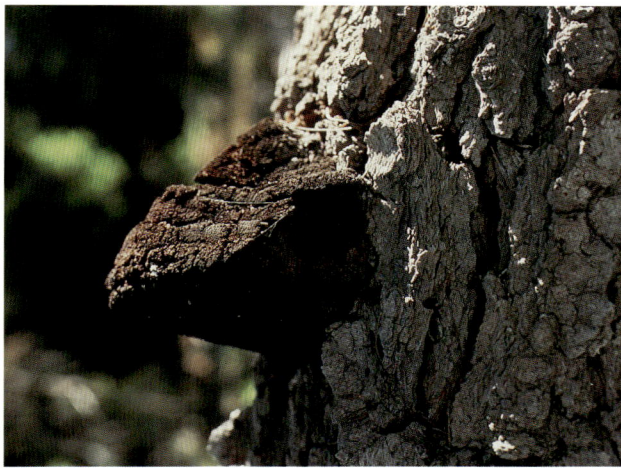

Figure 7-12— *Black, woody fruiting body of the Indian paint fungus on white fir.*

common on true firs in California, Oregon, and Washington and on hemlock in the Pacific Northwest and is considered a damaging butt rot organism in old-growth stands. The fungus commonly enters through fresh stumps, fire scars, dead or broken tops, and other wounds. The rot column, although usually in the butt and root systems, may occur anywhere in the heartwood. The fungus spreads from one tree to another by root grafting or from infected roots contacting non-infected roots. Long-distance spread is by spores infecting freshly cut stumps or wounded trees.

Field identification—

Rot—Incipient decay from annosus root and butt rot is not readily recognized. Discoloration may or may not be present, and heartwood remains firm and hard. In true firs and hemlock, incipient decay may appear as a reddish discoloration in the heartwood. In the advanced stage, the decayed wood is white, spongy, and may contain elongated white pockets (fig. 6-2). In true firs, the decayed wood often delaminates along the annual growth rings. No rhizomorphs are formed as they are in *Armillaria ostoyae*.

Fruiting body—The fruiting bodies of *H. annosum* vary considerably in shape and size. Their shape is indefinite. On pines they may appear as small, round, button-shaped structures growing under or protruding from the bark at the base of trees or less often as irregularly shaped, bracketlike bodies on the butts and roots of trees or within the wood of decaying stumps. Often they occur deep within hollow stumps of true firs and may develop to become almost a foot in width. When fresh, they are dark brown to gray on the upper surface and creamy white to pale orange on the lower pore surface (fig. 6-1).

Juniper Pocket Rot
Pyrofomes demidoffii (Fomes juniperinus)

Hosts—Western junipers are the known hosts.

Distribution and damage—This fungus is found on western juniper throughout its natural range in the western United States. The extent of decay in juniper stands throughout the Far West is not known. However, studies in stands of western juniper in Modoc County, CA, have shown that about 40 percent of the trees 12 inches (30 cm) and greater in basal diameter were infected with juniper pocket rot. Consequently, utilization of western juniper for pencil stock is uneconomical.

Field identification—

Rot—Juniper pocket rot may occur as either a butt or a trunk rot, depending on where the fungus entered the tree. Incipient decay first appears as a yellowish discoloration. Wood with advanced decay contains numerous large pockets lined with yellowish white fibers, and fungus mats and strands. These pockets often join to form fairly long tubes of stringy rot.

Fruiting body—Fruiting bodies are fairly common in the far western United States and when present indicate extensive heart rot. The upper surface of the woody hoof-shaped fruiting bodies is dark brown to nearly black and usually contains numerous deep cracks. The lower pore surface is light brown, and the interior is reddish brown.

Red Ring Rot/White Pocket Rot
Phellinus pini (Fomes pini)

Hosts—Douglas-fir, pines, true firs, larch, spruce, hemlock, western redcedar, and rarely incense-cedar are the known hosts.

Distribution and damage—Red ring rot occurs throughout the coniferous forests of the world, and in western North America is considered to be the single most damaging heart rot organism. Coastal Douglas-fir is the tree most commonly infected. Other coniferous tree species along the coast as well as conifers in the mountains of the West are also attacked. Millions of board feet of timber a year are lost or degraded as a result of rot caused by this organism. Red ring rot attacks second-growth as well as old-growth trees. Nearly all infections become established through living and dead branches or branch stubs. Open wounds rarely act as entrance points for this fungus. Thus, red ring rot may be one of the most serious heart rot problems in future forest stands.

Field identification—

Rot—Incipient decay appears as a discoloration of the heartwood. In pines, a pink to reddish color is present. Pronounced reddish-purple to olive discoloration appears in Douglas-fir.

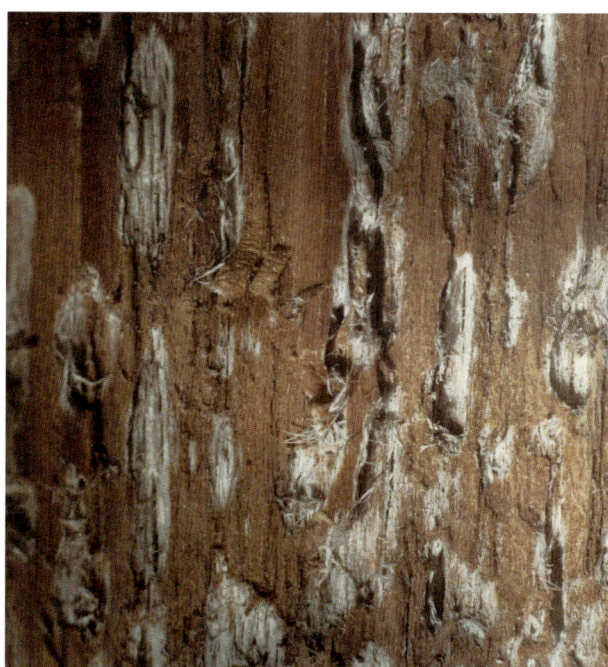

Figure 7-13—
White pocket rot of Douglas-fir caused by the red ring rot fungus (Phellinus pini).

Wood with advanced decay is often reddish and contains sharply margined small spindle-shaped pockets containing white, soft fibers (fig. 7-13). Mostly heartwood is affected, but sapwood is also invaded. Dark zone lines may also be observed in decayed wood. In cross section, the pockets may be evenly distributed throughout the wood (soft pines) or appear in rings (Douglas-fir, hard pines). The ring-like pattern of decay of heartwood is the result of the fungus attacking certain groups of annual rings and more readily destroying early wood rather than late wood. Swollen knots and punk knots are often indicators of decay by red ring rot.

Fruiting body—The perennial, woody fruiting bodies are the best indicators of decay. But they vary considerably in size, shape, and texture. One should be aware of this variability in identifying *Phellinus pini.* Fruiting bodies may range from about 2 to 10 inches (5 to 25 cm) in width and be thin and bracket-like or thick and hoof-shaped (fig. 7-14). The lower pore surface is usually a rich, rusty brown, the pores ranging from nearly round to maze-like. The upper surface is darker brown or dark gray and is usually marked with several concentric furrows.

Often a velvety margin separates the two surfaces. On living trees, the fruiting bodies nearly always arise from knots or branch

Figure 7-14—
Typical bracket-like fruiting bodies of red ring rot on Douglas-fir.

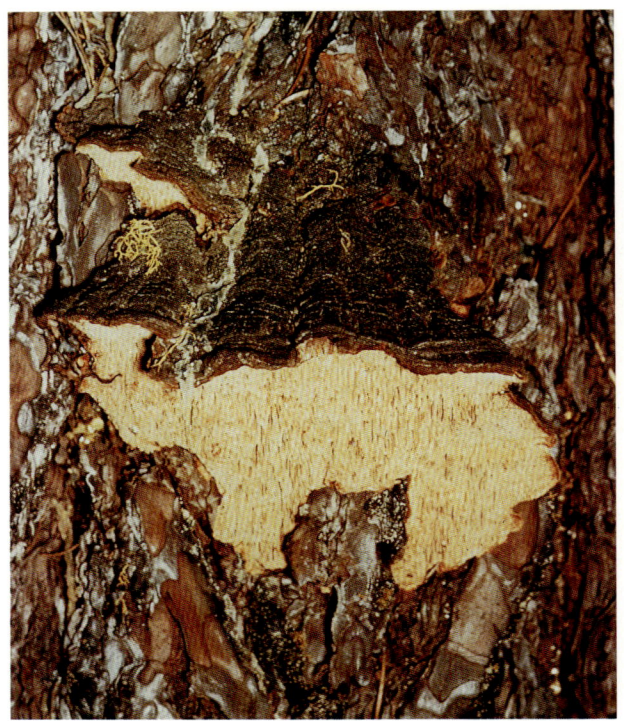

stubs. Sometimes only punk knots bearing the inner portion of the fruiting body remain on the tree. These punk knots may subsequently become overgrown with new wood. In these cases the swollen knots become the only symptom of decay.

Coral Fungus
Yellow Pitted Rot
Hericium abietis

Hosts—True firs, Engelmann spruce, and hemlock are common hosts.

Distribution and damage—This fungus is an important decay organism of true firs and hemlock in the Pacific Northwest, particularly in the Olympic Peninsula of Washington and in the mountains of eastern Oregon and Washington. It also occurs in the Rocky Mountains and in northern California. The rot may develop in the butt or upper portions of living trees, or in stumps, fallen trees, and snags. The coral fungus probably enters living trees through wounds and dead branches.

Field identification—

Rot—The advanced stage of this rot is similar to that caused by red ring rot, but the decayed wood is more yellowish. The elongate

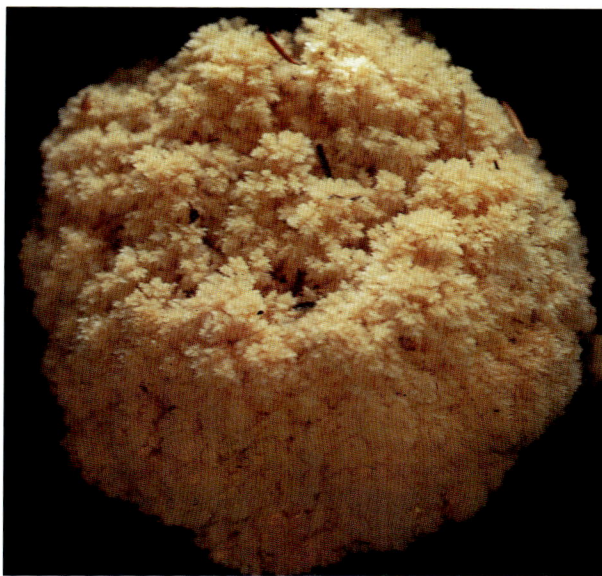

Figure 7-15—
*Fruiting body of the coral fungus (*Hericium abietis*) the cause of yellow pitted rot of true firs and hemlock.*

pockets formed in the wood are empty of noticeable white fibers. The color of the wood does not change noticeably.

Fruiting body—The fruiting bodies are soft, creamy white, corallike, and characterized mainly by the presence of numerous "spines," or "teeth," which produce spores (fig. 7-15). The fruiting bodies are short-lived and not readily recognized when shriveled and dry. They frequently appear near wounds.

Laminated Root Rot
Phellinus weirii

Hosts—In the Pacific Northwest, Douglas-fir, western hemlock, and western larch are the conifer species most frequently damaged. Farther east in the inland regions, western redcedar often suffers butt decay. For additional hosts attacked, see chapter 6 on root disease.

Distribution and damage—This fungus occurs throughout the Pacific Northwest from Northwestern California to British Columbia. *Phellinus weirii* is known mainly as a root disease organism (Chapter 6), but it does decay tree roots and butts. Heavy losses occur not only from tree mortality but also from blowdown as a result of root decay (fig. 7-16b).

Field identification—

Rot—Early decay by this organism appears as a red-brown stain in the outer heartwood. As the decay develops, the wood softens, small pits appear, and the annual rings separate to form the charac-

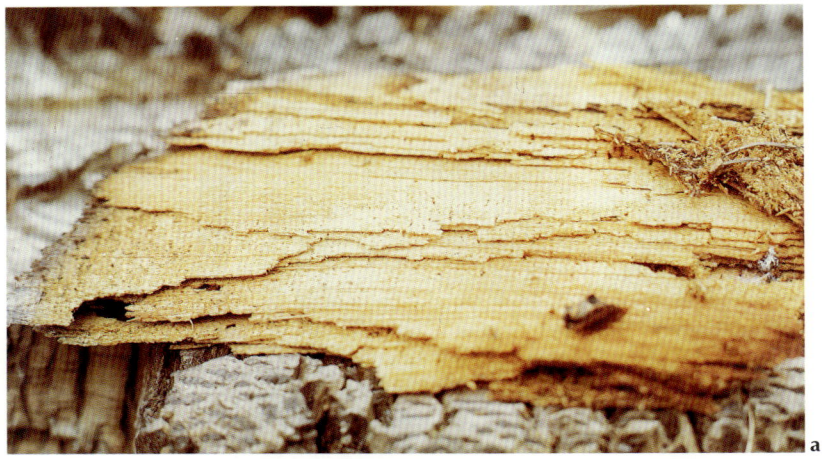

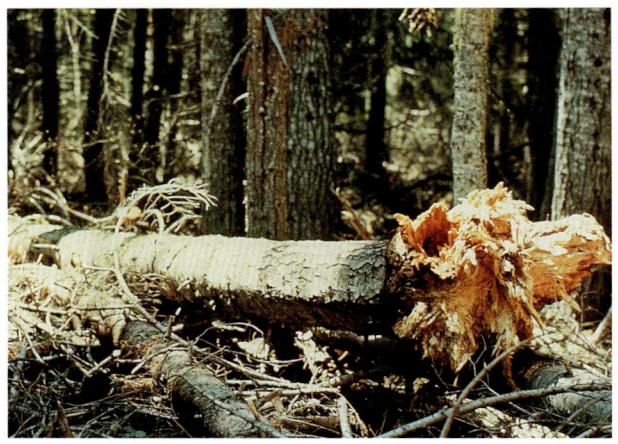

Figure 7-16—
Laminated root rot of Douglas-fir caused by Phellinus weirii *(**a**). Laminated root rot was responsible for the severe root decay of this wind-thrown Douglas-fir (**b**).*

teristic laminated rot (fig. 7-16a). At this stage the rotted wood is yellow to buff colored with dark brown mycelial felts often found between the laminations and in shrinkage cracks.

Fruiting body—For a description of the fruiting body, see chapter 6 on root disease.

Yellow Cap Fungus
Mottled Rot
Pholiota adiposa

Hosts—The hosts are true firs, pines, hemlock, and spruce.

Distribution and damage—This fungus is found on both hardwoods and conifers in the United States, but in the West, it is primarily a problem on true firs and hemlock. In California and parts of Oregon, it is considered a major heart rot organism in old-growth true fir stands. Young, unwounded trees are seldom infected. Fire scars, other basal wounds, frost cracks, and dwarf mistletoe bole cankers are the sites of infection for mottled rot. As a result, most of the rot occurs in the lower bole but has been found to extend 50 to 60 feet (15 to 19 m) above the ground.

Field identification—

Rot—The fungus produces a mottled appearance in the wood in the advanced stage of rot. Early decay appears as a light-cream to yellowish discoloration in heartwood. As the rot progresses, the areas darken and brownish streaks develop, forming small, widely scattered holes or pockets resembling insect burrows.

Yellowish-brown fungus strands fill the holes and shrinkage cracks. These strands may be best observed if the wood is split along the grain. Older trees with decay of long standing usually have a hollow butt.

Fruiting body—Other than shoestring root rot, mottled rot is the only major white rot of conifers caused by a gill-bearing, mushroom-like fungus (fig. 7-17). The yellow cap fungus fruits in the fall, usually after the first rains. The fresh fruiting structures consist of a yellowish central stalk and a cap that varies from yellow to yellowish brown on

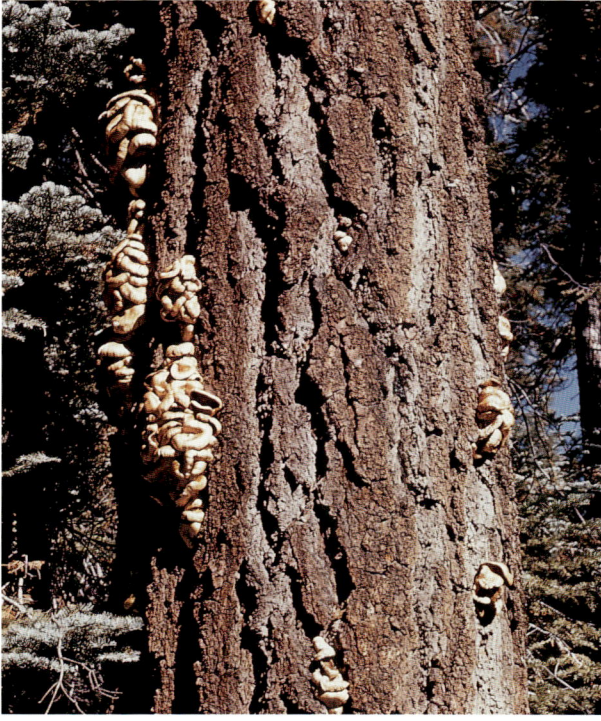

Figure 7-17— *Mushroom-like fruiting bodies of the yellow cap fungus (*Pholiota adiposa*) on white fir.*

the upper surface and yellow on the lower gill surface. The tops of the caps are sticky and slightly scaly. The mushrooms often occur in clusters and may appear on the trunk or from the base of infected trees. They are also commonly seen on stumps, down trees, and on the ends of cull logs. Old fruiting bodies dry and shrivel and turn black. They often persist for a year or more in this condition.

False Velvet Top Fungus
Red Root and Butt Rot
Inonotus tomentosus (Polyporus tomentosus)

Hosts—Pines, spruce, larch, hemlock, Douglas-fir, and true firs are known hosts; commonly observed on Engelmann spruce.

Distribution and damage—The fungus occurs on conifers throughout western North America but is most commonly found on hosts in the Pacific Northwest, British Columbia, and the Rocky Mountains. It appears to be found less often in the drier, arid regions of the Pacific Southwest.

Field identification—

Rot—The advanced stage of this rot closely resembles that of red ring rot. Many narrow pockets filled with white fibers occur in the heartwood. Affected wood usually becomes stained dark reddish brown to tan but retains its structural integrity as in the case with wood affected by red ring rot. This fungus primarily causes a root and butt rot and is seldom found more than a few feet above the ground in tree trunks.

Fruiting body—The fruiting bodies of this fungus resemble those produced by the velvet top fungus but are much smaller (usually about 2 to 3 inches (5 to 8 cm) in diameter) and lighter in color. The upper surface is yellow-brown to tan, zonate and slightly hairy in texture. The lower surface contains pores and is usually light brown. The fruiting bodies almost always occur on the ground in small clusters, where they arise from diseased roots. Occasionally they occur at the base of a tree.

White Ring Rot
Ceriporiopsis rivulosa (Poria albipellucida)

Hosts—The only hosts are coast redwood and western redcedar.

Distribution and damage—Except for brown cubical rot, white ring rot is the only other rot of any consequence associated with native stands of redwood. Whereas brown cubical rot is fairly evenly distributed throughout the natural range of redwood, white ring rot increases in severity from south to north. For instance, less than 10 percent of old-growth trees in Sonoma County, CA, were attacked by this fungus, but in Del Norte County, CA, nearly 75 percent of old-growth trees contained white ring rot. Western redcedar along the Pacific Coast is also often attacked by this fungus, and it is believed that the incidence of rot in redwood is correlated with the amount of western redcedar in the stand. Entrance courts for this fungus are wounds, mainly fire scars and dead or broken tops. Like brown cubical rot of redwood, white ring rot does not move into stump sprouts from rotted stumps.

Field identification—

Rot—Incipient rot looks like normal heartwood except for a dark brown discoloration. As the decay progresses, the heartwood softens and turns lighter brown. Wood with advanced decay is soft and cinnamon brown and often separates along the annual rings. Minute, elongated pits occur in the wood surfaces between these separations. These pitted surfaces may become somewhat hairy with whitish wood fibers as the rot continues. Wood in the final stage of decay appears as a stringy, fibrous mass.

Fruiting body—Fruiting bodies of this organism have never been found associated with decayed wood of redwood. The fungus was identified solely from laboratory cultures obtained from rotted wood. Fruiting bodies are found on western red cedar slash in the Pacific Northwest.

HEART ROT FUNGI OF MINOR IMPORTANCE

Fomitopsis cajanderi (Fomes subroseus), the cause of brown top rot in Douglas-fir, true fir, spruce, and some pines, occurs occasionally in northwestern California and in the Pacific Northwest. As the name implies, the rot often occurs in the uppermost part of the bole. This fungus is most common on dead trees and wood in service but can cause a brown cubical rot in the heartwood of Douglas-fir. Wood in the advanced stage of decay is soft, yellow to yellowish brown, and breaks into irregularly shaped cubes. The fruiting bodies are bracket like and woody, and have a pinkish rose lower pore surface and a rough, black-zoned upper surface (fig. 7-18).

Oligoporus balsameus (Polyporus basilaris) causes a brown cubical pocket rot in the butts of Monterey cypress (*Cupressus macrocarpa*). It occurs in natural stands in California and nearly everywhere Monterey cypress has been planted along the Pacific Coast. Trees 65 years and older are highly defective; 80 percent and more have rot. Trees less than 26 years old are practically rot-free. One to several fruiting bodies may be present, and these usually arise from branch stubs. Entrance of the fungus is thought to be through dead branches. Fruiting bodies are usually small (1 to 2 inches (3 to 6 cm) across), leathery, and bracketlike and vary from grayish brown to black.

Ganoderma oregonense, commonly called the lacquer fungus because of the shiny, reddish, lacquer-like upper surface of the

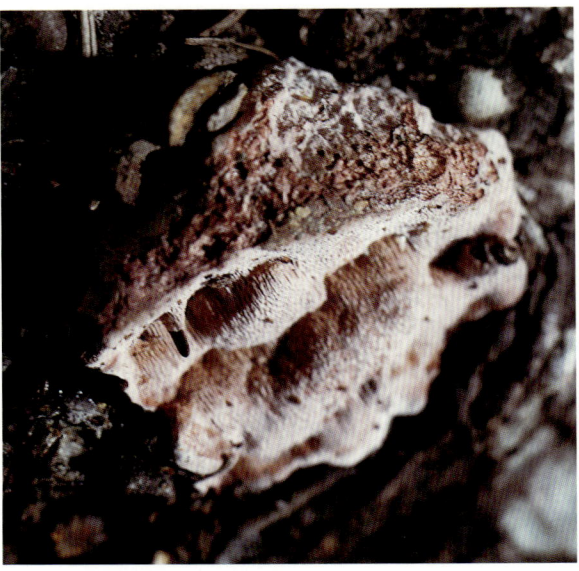

Figure 7-18—*Fruiting body of* Fomitopsis cajanderi, *the brown top rot fungus.*

fruiting body, decays primarily dead timber but occasionally causes a soft, spongy white rot of living trees (fig. 7-19). Decay in living trees is usually associated with wounds. The distinctive annual, bracket-type fruiting bodies have a cream-colored lower pore surface, are produced in the fall and often grow to be a foot or more across (fig. 7-20). The lacquer fungus attacks Douglas-fir, spruce, hemlock, and some pines along the Pacific Coast, and true firs throughout their natural range in California. Red fir is the most commonly attacked fir species.

Pleurotus ostreatus, the oyster mushroom, occasionally causes a white, flaky rot of the sapwood and heartwood of conifers in the western United States, but is most common on hardwoods. Infection usually occurs through open wounds, and the fungus has been observed invading true firs at the site of old, open bole infections of dwarf mistletoe. The white, fleshy, shelf-like mushrooms are smooth on their upper surface with gills on the lower surface, and often arise in clusters. The gills characteristically extend down along the stalk.

Cryptoporus volvatus (Polyporus volvatus), the pouch fungus, is not a heart-rotting fungus but causes a grayish white rot of the sapwood of most conifers in western North America. It is included only because it occurs so frequently in the forest and is often mistaken for a heart rot organism. For the most part, it occurs only on dead trees and snags within 1 to 2 years after the tree's death, but it has been observed on dead portions of living trees and on Douglas-fir weakened by bark beetles. The small, leathery, white fruiting bodies are produced in abundance within a short time after the tree is

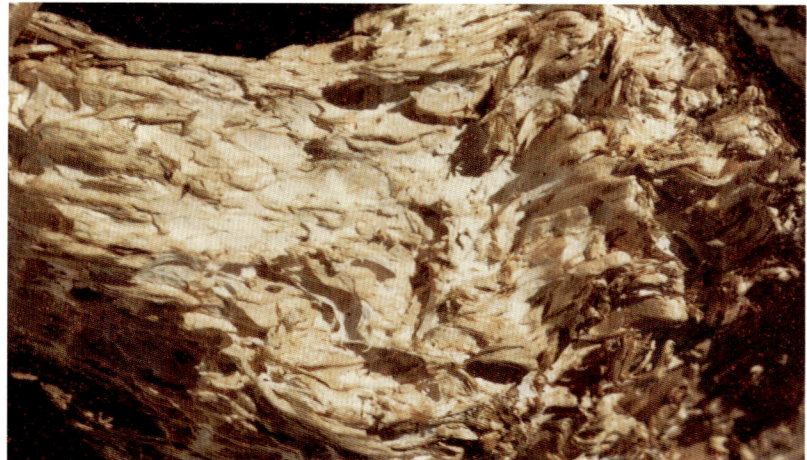

Figure 7-19—*White spongy rot of red fir caused by the lacquer fungus* (Ganoderma oregonense).

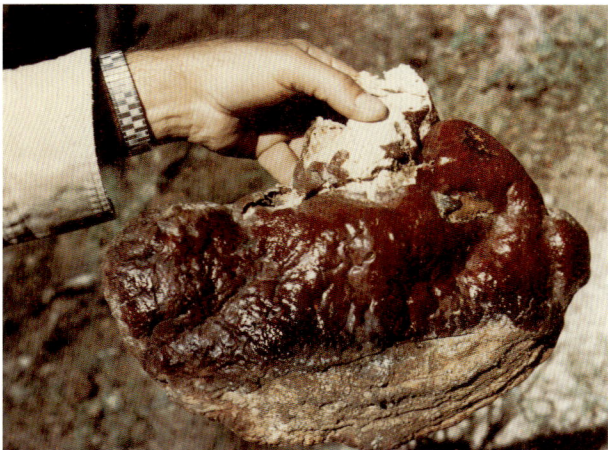

Figure 7-20—*The lacquer fungus produces large distinctive fruiting bodies.*

attacked (fig. 7-21). One of their distinguishing features is the lower spore-bearing surface that is covered by a fungus sheath except for a single hole through which insects enter, feed, and then exit and move on to spread the fungus. This unique adaptation to spread by beetles and other insects accounts for the rapidity with which it invades dead and dying trees.

Dichomitus squalens (Polyporus anceps) or red rot often occurs in ponderosa, Jeffrey, and Coulter pines in southern California. It is rare elsewhere along the Pacific Coast, but is common and damaging on pines in the Southwest and Rocky Mountains. This fungus acts both as a decomposer of dead wood and as a heart rot. In living

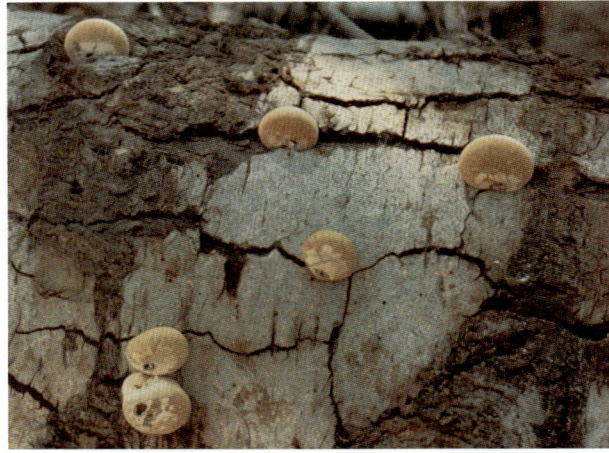

Figure 7-21—
*Small, leathery fruiting bodies of the pouch fungus (*Cryptoporus volvatus*) occur on a white fir log.*

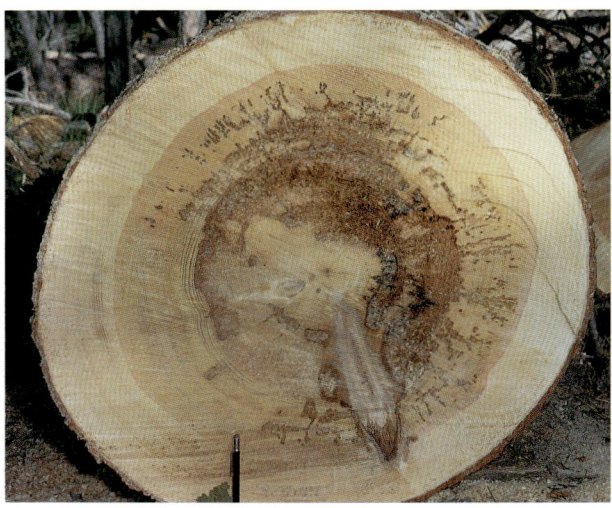

Figure 7-22—
*Decay of ponderosa pine caused by red rot (*Dichomitus squalens*).*

trees, the fungus frequently enters through broken tops, causing considerable rot of the upper boles. It can also enter through bole wounds and large dead limbs. Advanced decay is a white pocket rot—not unlike that caused by the red ring rot organism *Phellinus pini* (fig. 7-22). Wood infected by red rot does not remain firm but tends to crumble and disintegrate when handled. Fruiting bodies are rarely found on living trees but occur mostly on the underside of down logs or on slash. They appear as white to light brown crusts of irregular shape on down trunks and branches. Detection of the rot in living trees is difficult.

Ganoderma applanatum, commonly called the artists' fungus, is the cause of white mottled rot of several conifers, especially Douglas-

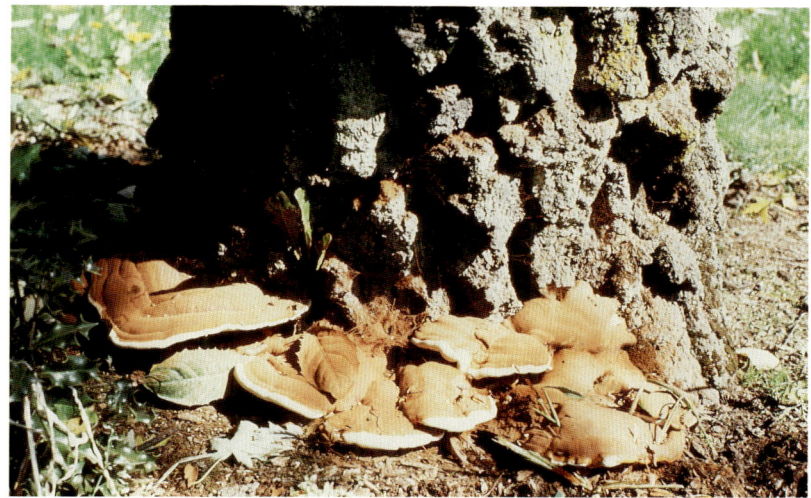

Figure 7-23—*Fresh fruiting bodies of the artists' fungus* (Ganoderma applanatum) *growing from the base of an old birch tree.*

fir and western hemlock. *G. applanatum* is common throughout western Oregon, Washington, and British Columbia. Though especially common on living or dead hardwoods, it also causes white mottled rot of conifers. It is often found decaying dead conifers and occasionally rots heartwood and living sapwood of wounded Douglas-fir and western hemlock. *G. applanatum* spreads by windborne spores. Infection of living trees apparently occurs through wounds, especially sizable trunk wounds and large broken tops on decadent, old trees. *G. applanatum* causes a spongy, mottled white rot with many fine, black zone lines. It produces hard, woody, shelf-like perennial conks that may reach a width of 2 feet (0.6 m) or more. The upper surfaces are smooth and tan to dark brown (fig. 7-23). The undersurface is white to yellowish and turns brown when bruised or scratched.

Perenniphoria subacida, the cause of yellow root rot of hemlock, Douglas-fir, lodgepole pine, western larch, grand fir, and western redcedar occurs throughout the Pacific Northwest. It causes a root and butt rot of suppressed or weakened trees and is a common saprophyte of dead trees. Vigorous trees are rarely affected. Incipient decay caused by *P. subacida* looks like wetwood. Advanced decay is a yellow-white, spongy rot. The annual rings of decayed wood separate easily, and the decay is sometimes confused with laminated root rot. However, *P. subacida* decay lacks pitting in the decayed wood layers. Fruiting bodies are crustlike, appressed, up to 0.5 inch (1.3 cm) thick, and 2 to 3 feet (0.6 to 0.9 m) long. They are white when fresh, becoming creamy to yellow orange with age. Conks are usually found on undersides of logs, fallen trees, exposed roots, and undersides of root crotches. Spread appears to involve growth from tree to tree via root contacts rather than spore spread.

SELECTED REFERENCES

Bailey, H.B. 1941. The biology of *Polyporus basilarus*. Torrey Botanical Club Bulletin 68:112–120.
Boyce, John Shaw. 1961. Forest pathology. 3d ed., New York: McGraw-Hill. 572 p.
Etheridge, D.H.; Craig, H.M.; Parris, S.H. 1972. Infection of western hemlock by the Indian paint fungus via living branches. Environment Canada, Forestry Service Bimonthly Research Note 28:3–4.
Fritz, Emanual; Bonar, Lee. 1931. The brown heart rot of California redwood. Journal Forestry 29(3):368–380.
Gilbertson, R.L.; Ryvarden, L. 1986. North American polypores. Fungiflora. Oslo, Norway: A/S/. 885 p.
Hadfield, James S.; Johnson, David W. 1977. Laminated root rot: a guide for reducing and preventing losses in Oregon and Washington forests. Res. Bull. Portland, OR: U.S. Department of Agriculture, Forest Service, Pacific Northwest Region. 16 p.
Kimmey, James W. 1950. Cull factors for forest tree species in northwestern California. Surv. Rel. 7. Berkeley, CA: U.S. Department of Agriculture, Forest Service, Calif. Forest and Range Experiment Station. 30 p.
Kimmey, James W. 1955. The heart rots of redwood. For. Pest Leafl. 25. Washington, DC: U.S. Department of Agriculture. 4 p.
Kimmey, James W. 1965. Rust-red stringy rot. For. Pest Leafl. 93. Washington, DC: U.S. Department of Agriculture. 8 p.
Kimmey, James W.; Bynum, H.H. 1961. Heart rots of red and white firs. For. Pest Leafl. 52. Washington, DC: U.S. Department of Agriculture. 4 p.
Kimmey, James W.; Lightle, Paul C. 1955. Fungi associated with cull in redwood. Forest Science 1(2):104–110.
Meinecke, E.P. 1914. Forest tree diseases common in California and Nevada. A manual for field use. Washington, DC: U.S. Department of Agriculture, Forest Service. 67 p.
Partridge, Arthur D.; Miller, Daniel L. 1974. Major decays of wood in the Inland Northwest. Univ. Nat. Resources Ser., No. 3. Moscow, ID: Idaho Research Foundation, Inc. 125 p.
Wagener, W.W. 1929. *Lentinus lepideus* Fr.: a cause of heart rot of living trees. Phytopathology 19:705–712.
Wagener, Willis W.; Bega, Robert V. 1958. Heart rots of incense-cedar. For. Pest Leafl. 30. Washington, DC: U.S. Department of Agriculture. 7 p.
Wagener, Willis W.; Davidson, Ross W. 1954. Heart rots in living trees. Botanical Review 20:61–131.

Glossary

Aerial shoot—stem-like portion of dwarf mistletoe outside the host bark stem whose primary function is to reproduce.

Alternate host—one or the other of two unlike hosts of a heteroecious fungus, i.e., some rust fungi.

Annual canker—a canker that occurs only during one period of time of the year or season, usually caused by adverse environmental conditions or organisms.

Annulus—a ring of fungus tissue encircling the stem of some mushrooms, as in the shoestring fungus.

Apothecium, apothecia—a cup- or saucer-like sexual fruiting body which produces ascospores.

Appressed—pressed close to the surface, as against the bark of a tree.

Ascocarp—a sexual or perfect fruiting body of the Ascomycete, which produces its spores within an ascus.

Ascospores—a spore produced in an ascus (see ascus).

Ascus, asci—a sac-like cell of the perfect stage of the Ascomycete in which ascospores—usually eight—are produced.

Asexual stage—a stage in the life cycle of a fungus in which spores are produced without a previous sexual fusion; (synonym: imperfect stage).

Autoecious—a fungus that completes its life cycle on one host, for example, some rust fungi.

Basal cup—the cup-like remnant on the bark of a branch infected by dwarf mistletoe that remains visible long after the disintegration of an aerial shoot.

Basal shoot scar—see basal cup.

Biotic factors—the living organisms in an ecosystem and their relationship with other organisms.

Bicolor—two colors (relating to the fruit of dwarf mistletoe that are bicolor).

Blight—a loose term for a disease causing rapid death or dieback.

Bole—a tree stem once it has grown to substantial thickness—roughly capable of yielding saw timber; similar to trunk stem.

Bracket-type fungus—laterally attached, shelf-like fungal fruiting bodies occurring on trees; mostly of the wood decay type.

Broom—see witches-broom.

Brown rot—a light to dark brown decay of wood that is friable and rectangularly checked in the advanced stage, caused by fungi that attack mainly the cellulose and associated carbohydrates; residue is chiefly lignin.

Burl—a hard, woody, abnormal outgrowth in a tree, more or less rounded in form. Usually resulting from the entwined growth of a cluster of adventitious buds, sometimes from an old wound.
Butt rot—a rot characteristically confined to the butt or lower trunk of a tree.

Canker—a definite, relatively localized, necrotic lesion primarily of the bark and cambium.
Cellulose—a complex carbohydrate occurring in most all plant material; a major component of wood.
Colonize—to establish an infection within a host or part of a host.
Concolorous—of the same color.
Confluent—running into one another, merging.
Conk—the large, often bracket-like fruiting bodies of wood-destroying fungi (Basidiomycetes).
Cubical cracking—the characteristic of woods in an advanced stage of brown rot; to break up into distinct cubes.
Cull factor—a calculated percentage of the amount of merchantable wood lost from a tree as a result of decay or other defect.
Decay—the decomposition of wood by fungi.
Decline—the gradual reduction in health and vigor as a tree is in the process of dying slowly.
Decomposer—organism that physically and chemically breaks down dead organisms into simpler compounds and elements.
Defect—any imperfection in a tree that reduces the volume of sound wood or lowers its durability, strength, or utility.
Dieback—the progressive dying, from the tip downward, of twigs, branches, or tops.
Discoloration—a change in hue or color.
Disease—the alteration of the function or the form of a plant from normal.
Disease cycle—the chain of events in the development of a disease.
Dry rot—a decay of the brown rot type, caused by specialized fungi able to conduct moisture from an available source and extend their attack to wood previously too dry to decay.
Duff—the litter and partially decomposed litter on the forest floor.

Early wood—the less dense, larger—celled portion of an annual growth ring formed during the early part of the growing season.
Elliptical—shaped like an ellipse, oblong with regularly rounded ends.
Endemic—a disease that is at its usual normal balanced level within a region to which it is indigenous; not epidemic or rampant.
Entrance court—the point of invasion of a disease organism into its host.

Environment—the sum total of all the biotic (living) and abiotic (non- living) factors affecting an individual's surroundings.
Epidemic—a disease that occurs periodically, widely, and rapidly, and reaches injurious levels.
Exudate—matter that oozes out or is secreted out.

Facultative parasite—an organism normally saprophytic but capable of changing to a parasitic life.
Fade—to change foliage color slightly in the early process of dying; usually changes occur from a dark green toward a lighter gray-green.
Flagging—displaying dead brown branches known as flags among the rest of the living crown.
Flags—conspicuous dead branches with foliage remaining as a result of rapid killing by adverse abiotic conditions or disease agents.
Form—a description below the subspecies or variety level but is still distinguishable morphologically.
Fruiting body—any of a number of kinds of reproductive structures that produces spores.
Fungus—one of a group of organisms considered by some authorities to be lower plants that lack chlorophyll.
Fungus mat—dense, leathery mass of fungus mycelium often formed in decayed wood by certain wood rotting fungi.
Fusiform swelling—a swelling on a host branch or stem that is typically widest near the middle and tapers toward each end (synonym: spindle-shaped swelling).

Galls—pronounced swellings on woody plants caused by certain insects and disease organisms.
Germinate—the beginning of growth by a seed or spore.
Gill fungi—those fungi with mushroom-shaped fruiting bodies that bear gill-like plates on the underside of the cap.
Gills—blade-like, spore-bearing structures on the lower surface of the fruiting bodies of certain fungi.
Globose—spherical.

Hard pine—any pines of the subgenus *Pinus* (Diploxylon).
Heart rot—a decay characteristically confined to the heartwood.
Heartwood—the inner layers of wood that, in the growing tree, have ceased to contain living cells and in which the reserve materials (for example, starch and sugars) have been removed or converted into more durable substances.
Heteroecious—a fungus that must pass different stages of its life cycle on unlike hosts, that is, some rust fungi.

Hoof-shaped—appearing like a hoof; for example, the bracket-type fruiting bodies of certain wood decay fungi that are flat on the bottom and rounded on the sides and top.
Host—the plant on or in which a pathogen exists.
Host range—all the hosts that a particular pathogen attacks.
Host specific—disease organisms that attack only certain species of hosts.
Hysterothecium, hysterothecia—a specialized fruiting body of needle cast fungi that is usually elongate and covered and opens at maturity by a long slit.

Immune—unable to be attacked by an organism.
Incidence—rate of occurrence.
Incipient decay, incipient rot—the early stage of wood decay in which the wood is invaded and may show discoloration but is not otherwise visibly altered.
Infection—the act of a pathogen establishing itself on or within a host.
Infection site—the area in which the pathogen first established itself on or in the host.
Infest—to be present in such numbers within an area as to be a source of danger.
Inner bark—the active layer of tissues (phloem and cambium) between the wood (xylem) and the suberized bark.
Inoculum—the spores or tissues of a pathogen that infect a host or crop.
Inoculum potential—the general mass of the pathogen (including spores and tissues) and its relative virulence which are available for infection.

Late wood—the denser, smaller celled portion of an annual growth ring formed during the latter part of the growing season.
Life cycle—in fungi, the stage or series of stages between one spore form and the development of the same spore again.
Lignin—a substance impregnating the cell wall in woody tissue; along with cellulose, it is the principal component of wood.
Litter—see duff.

Microsclerotium—a tiny (microscopic) sclerotium.
Mortality—death from disease.
Mycelial fans—similar in structure to mycelial felts but fan-shaped.
Mycelial felt—a mass of fungus filaments arranged in a flat plane that resemble a thin felt-like paper or cloth.
Mycelial pads—small mats of compacted mycelia that are often formed by fungi on or in the host.

Mycelial strands—a mass or group of fungus filaments that appear as visible strands to the naked eye.
Mycelium, mycelia—a mass of hyphae that forms the vegetative filamentous body of a fungus.

Necrosis—death of plant cells usually resulting in darkening of the tissue.
Necrotic spot (area)—a dead area on a living plant; often caused by biotic and abiotic diseases.
Needle cast—a disease of needles of conifers caused by a group of fungi in the family Rhytismataceae.
Needle complement—the normal or usual number of needles that a conifer of a particular species will bear.
Needle spotting—a needle disease characterized by isolated circular or elongate lesions.

Obligate parasite—a parasite incapable of existing independently of live host tissue.

Parasite—an organism living on and nourished by another living organism.
Parasitic—living on or in another organism and deriving nourishment therefrom.
Pathogen—an organism that causes a disease.
Pendant—hanging, pendulous.
Perennial—continuing growth from year to year.
Perennial canker—the recurrent yearly killing back and healing over of the bark and cambial tissue of woody plants by certain disease organisms.
Perithecium, perithecia—a closed, flask-like sexual fruiting body produced by certain Ascomycetes containing asci and ascospores.
Pocket rot—a characteristic pattern of rot caused by certain fungi; the rot occurs in distinct, scattered pockets within the heartwood of a tree rather than in a distinct column.
Pore surface—the surface of the fruiting body of certain wood-decaying fungi (Polyporaceae) that consists of small openings or pores.
Predispose—to make susceptible.
Predisposition—the effect of environmental and biotic factors that make a plant vulnerable to attack by a pathogen.
Primary host—see principal host.
Principal host—the main host for a particular disease organism; used particularly regarding the main host species infected by dwarf mistletoes.

Punk knot—soft, decayed branch stubs that usually indicate the presence of decay in a tree.
Pustule—blisters caused by certain disease fungi, often maturing into the spore-bearing structures of the disease organism.
Pycnidium, pycnidia—an asexual type of fruiting body, typically flask-like, that produces asexual spores or conidia.

Resinosis—the unnatural and profuse flow or accumulation of resin from conifers injured or attacked by insects and disease.
Resistant—able to withstand without serious injury an attack by an organism or damage by a nonliving agent but not immune from such attacks.
Rhizomorph—a specialized thread or cord-like structure made up of parallel hyphae with a protective covering.
Root crown—the upper-most portion of the root system where the major roots join together at the base of the stem.
Root grafting—the union of the roots of two different trees as a result of physical contact.
Rot—the physical and chemical deterioration of wood caused by wood-rotting fungi.
Rot column—the vertical column of rotted wood within the heartwood of a tree invaded by heart rot fungi.

Saprophyte—an organism using dead organic material as food.
Sapwood—the outer conducting layers of wood, which in the growing tree contain living cells and reserve materials.
Secondary host—a host species attacked less commonly than the principal host.
Sexual stage—the stage in the life cycle of a fungus in which spores are formed after sexual fusion (synonym: perfect stage).
Scale-like leaves—a scale-like structure that is morphologically a leaf often reduced in size (as bud scale, various bracts).
Sclerotium—a firm, frequently rounded, often black mass of hyphae often acting as a resting body.
Shoot scar—see basal cup.
Shot hole—depression in the bark caused by woodpeckers searching for insects at the base of an old fruiting body (conk); indicator of decay.
Signs—visible evidence of the disease organism, fruiting bodies.
Soft pine—any pines of the subgenus *Strobus* (Haploxylon).
Spindle-shaped swelling—see fusiform swelling.
Spores—the final reproductive structure of the fungi and other lower plants.
Sporulation—the act of producing and liberating spores.

Stain—the dark brown to black discolorations of wood caused by the presence of certain fungi; not to be confused with wetwood.
Susceptible—unable to withstand attack by an organism or damage by a nonliving agent without serious injury.
Symptoms—the noticeable evidence of disturbances in the normal development and life processes of the host plant.

Teeth—see toothed surface.
Toothed surface—the tooth-like texture of the spore-bearing surface of certain wood decay fungi; for example, Indian paint fungus.

Upward spread—see vertical intensification.

Vertical intensification—the spread upward of dwarf mistletoe within a tree (synonym: upward spread).
Virulent—vigorously pathogenic.

Wetwood—a discolored, water-soaked condition of the heartwood of some conifers presumably caused by bacterial fermentation; often associated with distinctive odor, gas production, and an exudation called slime flux.
White rot—decay caused by fungi that attack all chief constituents of wood and leave a whitish or light colored residue; wood is often fibrous or spongy in texture.
Wilt—the collapse of a plant or part of a plant because of a loss of cell turgidity.
Witches-broom—an abnormally profuse, dense mass of host branches and foliage (synonym: broom).

Xerophytic—adapted to dry conditions.
Xylem—the woody tissue of the stem, branches, and roots.

Zone lines—narrow, dark brown or black lines in a decayed wood caused by fungi.

Index to Host Plants, With Scientific Names

Apple, *Malus* ssp.   104
Aster, *Aster* spp.   97

Bastard toadflax, *Comandra umbellata* Nutt.   93
Bearberry, *Arctostaphylos uva-ursi*   109
Blueberry, *Vaccinium* spp.   101

Chickweed, *Stellaria* spp.   98
Coast redwood, *Sequoia sempervirens* (D. Don) Endl.   4, 11, 16, 24, 78, 162, 174
Cypress Family, *Cupressaceae*   77, 115
    Arizona cypress, *Cupressus arizonica* Greene   13, 108–109
    Baker (Modoc) cypress, *Cupressus bakeri* Jeps.   108
    Gowan cypress, *Cupressus goveniana* Gord.   109
    Italian cypress, *Cupressus sempervirens* L.   13
    Monterey cypress, *Cupressus macrocarpa* Hartw.   16, 77, 175

Douglas-fir, *Pseudotsuga menziesii* (Mirb.) Franco   4–5, 7, 10–13, 23–24, 29–30, 39–40, 44, 67–70, 74, 80–81, 102, 127, 138, 141, 144, 146, 155, 158, 160, 162, 165, 168, 171, 174–179
    big-cone Douglas-fir, *Pseudotsuga macrocarpa* (Vasey) Mayr.   22, 40, 102

Figwort, *Scrophularia* spp.   89
Firs, *Abies* spp.   12, 66–68, 80, 101–102, 127, 138, 141, 147, 155, 158, 160, 162, 165, 168, 170, 172, 174–176
    bristlecone fir, *Abies bracteata* D. Don. ex Poiteau   44
    California red fir, *Abies magnifica* A. Murr.   22, 24, 42, 75, 98, 122
    grand fir, *Abies grandis* (Dougl. ex D. Don) Lindl.   4, 9, 23-24, 42, 44, 69, 75, 98, 122, 146, 179
    noble fir, *Abies procera* Rehd.   42, 133-134
    Pacific silver fir, *Abies amabilis* Dougl. ex Forbes   42, 75, 133–134
    subalpine fir, *Abies lasiocarpa* (Hook.) Nutt.   9, 23, 44, 75, 98, 134
    white fir, *Abies concolor* (Gord. & Glend.) Lindl. ex Hilderbr.   4–5, 7, 11, 13, 17, 22, 24–25, 29, 42, 44, 75–76, 98, 115, 122, 146

Goldenrod, *Solidago* spp.   97

Gooseberry (See *Ribes*)

Hawthorn, *Crataegus* spp.   104, 107, 108
Hemlock, *Tsuga* spp.   80, 138, 141, 144, 147, 155, 158, 160, 162, 165, 168, 170, 172, 174, 176, 179
   mountain hemlock, *Tsuga mertensiana* (Bong.) Carr.   133, 144
   western hemlock, *Tsuga heterophylla* (Raf.) Sarg.   23, 133, 144, 146, 155, 171, 178

Incense-cedar, *Libocedrus decurrens* Torr.   5, 9, 13, 17, 18, 22, 29, 36, 38, 65, 104, 117, 138, 141, 158–160, 168

Juniper, *Juniperus* spp.   11, 18, 23, 36, 77, 106, 115, 117, 138, 141
   alligator juniper, *Juniperus deppeana* Steud.   7
   California juniper, *Juniperus californica* Carr.   108
   oneseed juniper, *Juniperus monosperma* (Engelm.) Sarg.   107–108
   Rocky Mountain juniper, *Juniperus scopulorum* Sarg.   108
   Utah juniper, *Juniperus osteosperma* (Torr.) Little   107–108
   western juniper, *Juniperus occidentalis* Hook.   23, 107–108, 117, 168

Kinnikinnick, *Arctostaphylos uva-ursi*   109

Larch, *Larix* spp.   80, 160, 162, 168, 174
   western larch, *Larix occidentalis* Nutt.   23, 36, 128, 155, 171, 179

Mountain ash, *Sorbus* spp.   104
Mouse-ear chickweed, *Cerastium*   98

Pacific yew, *Taxus brevifolia* Nutt.   23
Paint brush, *Castilleja* sp.   89, 91
Pear, *Pyrus communis* L.   104, 106–107
Pines, *Pinus* spp.   34, 66, 68, 74, 92, 138, 141, 147, 155, 158, 160, 162, 168, 172, 174–176
   Aleppo pine, *Pinus halepensis* Miller   13, 73
   Apache pine, *Pinus engelmannii* Carr.   91
   bishop pine, *Pinus muricata* D. Don.   48, 73, 97, 130
   bristlecone pine, *Pinus aristata* Engelm.   85
   Coulter pine, *Pinus coulteri* D. Don.   4, 13, 22, 47, 54, 89, 97, 125, 131, 176
   Digger pine, *Pinus sabiniana* Dougl.   13, 17, 54, 124, 131
   eastern white pine, *Pinus strobus* L.   85
   foxtail pine, *Pinus balfouriana* Grev. & Balf.   85, 125
   Italian stone pine, *Pinus pinea* L.   13, 73

Jeffrey pine, *Pinus jeffreyi* Grevl. & Balf.   5, 13, 17, 20, 22, 47,
    54, 57–58, 66, 89, 91, 93, 97, 124, 132, 144, 176
knobcone pine, *Pinus attenuata* Lemm.   13, 22, 47–48, 54–56,
    93, 124, 131–132, 144
lodgepole pine, *Pinus contorta* Dougl. ex Loud.   5, 13, 15,
    23–24, 47–48, 54, 57–58, 63–64, 89, 92–93, 97–98,
    122, 130, 133, 144, 179
limber pine, *Pinus flexilis* James   7, 9, 51–52, 85, 125
Mexican white pine, *Pinus flexilis* var. *reflexa* Engelm.   85
Monterey X knobcone hybrid, *Pinus radiata x attenuata*   48
Monterey pine, *Pinus radiata* D. Don.   4, 11, 13, 18, 22, 48, 54,
    56, 58, 73, 92, 97, 130
pinyon, *Pinus edulis* Engelm.   47, 52, 95
ponderosa pine, *Pinus ponderosa* Dougl. ex Laws.   4, 5, 7, 11,
    13, 15, 20, 22–24, 27, 29, 47–48, 54–55, 57–58, 89,
    91–93, 122, 124, 132, 144, 176
Scotch pine, *Pinus sylvestris* L.   54, 93
singleleaf pinyon, *Pinus monophylla* Torr. & Frem.   13, 47, 52,
    95, 127, 144
sugar pine, *Pinus lambertiana* Dougl.   5, 13, 17–18, 22, 24, 29,
    50, 52, 54, 63, 85, 122–123, 131, 144
Torrey pine, *Pinus torreyana* Parry ex Carr.   13
western white pine, *Pinus monticola* Dougl. ex D. Don.   12–13,
    23–24, 48, 50–52, 54, 63, 85, 123, 125, 131, 133, 144
whitebark pine, *Pinus albicaulis* Engelm.   51–52, 54, 85, 125,
    134
Poplars, *Populus* spp.   103
Port-Orford-cedar, *Chamaecyparis lawsoniana* (A. Murr.) Parl.   148

Quince, *Cydonia* spp.   104, 107

Ribes, *Ribes* spp.   85, 95

Sequoia, *Sequoiadendron giganteum* (Lindl.) Buchholz   11, 24, 65,
    138
Serviceberry, *Amelanchier* spp.   104, 106–108
Singles delight, *Moneses uniflora*   109
Spruces, *Picea* spp.   12, 80, 109, 127, 138, 141, 147, 155, 160,
    162, 165, 168, 172, 174–176
  blue spruce, *Picea pungens* Engelm.   23
  Brewer spruce, *Picea brewerana* ats.   35, 122
  Engelmann spruce, *Picea engelmannii* Parry ex Engelm.   9, 23,
    35, 170
  Sitka spruce, *Picea sitchensis* (Bong.) Carr.   35
  white spruce, *Picea glauca* (Moench) Voss   23

Sweetfern, *Comptonia* spp.   97

Tarweed, *Hemizonia* spp., *Madia* spp.   97
Thuja, *Thuja* spp.   23, 80

Western redcedar, *Thuja plicata* Donn ex D. Don   9, 23–24, 138, 146, 155, 160, 162, 168, 171, 174, 179
Willow, *Salix* spp.   102
Wintergreen, *Pyrola* sp.   109

Index to Diseases and Causal Agents

Air pollutants   18
Amelanchier rust   106
Annosus root disease   138
Annosus root and butt rot   166
Arceuthobium abietinum   122
   (f.sp. *concoloris*)   122
   (f.sp. *magnificae*)   122
Arceuthobium americanum   123
Arceuthobium californicum   123
Arceuthobium campylopodum   124
Arceuthobium cyanocarpum   125
Arceuthobium divaricatum   127
Arceuthobium douglasii   127
Arceuthobium laricis   128
Arceuthobium littorum   130
Arceuthobium monticolum   131
Arceuthobium occidentale   125, 131
Arceuthobium siskiyouense   132
Arceuthobium tsugense subsp. *mertensianae*   133
Arceuthobium tsugense subsp. *tsugense*   133
Armillaria ostoyae   137, 141, 164
Armillaria root disease   141
Artists' fungus   178
Aster rust   97
Atropellis canker   63
Atropellis pinicola   63
Atropellis piniphila   64

Bacterial gall of Douglas-fir   81
Bark scorch   12
Bifusella linearis   51
Bifusella pini   52
Bifusella saccata   52
Black stain root disease   144
Bole injuries   29, 30
Borate damage (See herbicide toxicity)
Botryosphaeria canker of giant sequoia   65
Botryosphaeria ribis   65
Branch injuries   29, 30
Bristlecone fir needle cast   44
Brown crumbly rot   155
Brown cubical rot   162
Brown cubical rot of cypress   175

Brown felt blight   34
Brown stringy rot   165
Brown top rot   175
Brown trunk rot   155

Cedar leaf blight   38
Cenangium canker   66
Cenangium ferruginosum   66
Ceriporiopsis rivulosa   174
Charcoal root disease   149
Chlorate damage (See herbicide toxicity)
Chloride salt accumulation (See road salt damage)
Chloride ions   15
Chlorosis   18
Chlorotic mottle (See ozone damage)
Chronic ozone injury (See ozone damage)
Chrysomyxa arctostaphyli   109
Chrysomyxa monesis   109
Chrysomyxa pirolata   109
Coleosporium asterum   97
Coleosporium madiae   97
Coleosporium solidaginis   97
Commandra blister rust   93
Contact herbicides (See herbicide toxicity)
Coral fungus   170
Coryneum cardinale   77
Coastal dwarf mistletoe   130
Coastal spruce cone rust   109
Cronartium coleosporioides   89
Cronartium comandrae   93
Cronartium comptoniae   97
Cronartium occidentale   95
Cronartium ribicola   85
Cryptoporus volvatus   176
Cyclaneusma niveum   58
Cypress canker   77
Cypress-juniper mistletoe   115
Cytospora abietis   67, 122
Cytospora canker of true firs   67, 122

Dasyscyphus canker of conifers   68
Dasyscyphus sp.   68
Davisomycella lacrimiformis   56
Davisomycella limitata   56
Davisomycella medusa   57

Davisomycella montana 57
De-icing salt 15
Dense mistletoe 115
Dermea canker of Douglas-fir 69
Dermea pseudotsugae 69
Diaporthe lokoyae 70
Dichomitus squalens 177
Didymascella thujina 38
Digger pine dwarf mistletoe 131
Diplodia canker 74
Diplodia pinea 74
Dothistroma septospora 48
Douglas-fir dwarf mistletoe 127
Douglas-fir needle cast 40
Douglas-fir rust 102
Drooping needles 12
Drought damage 13
Dwarf mistletoe 118

Echinodontium tinctorium 165
Elytroderma deformans 47
Elytroderma disease 47
Excess fertilizer 17
Excess soil moisture 14

False velvet top fungus 174
Filamentosum rust 91
Fir blueberry rust 101
Fir needle casts 42
Fir willow weed rust 102
Fire damage 23
Fluorine (hydrogen fluoride) 23
Fomes annosus (See *Heterobasidion annosum*)
Fomes juniperinus 168
Fomes officinalis 155
Fomes pini 168
Fomes pinicola 155
Fomes root and butt rot 152–153, 166
Fomes subroseus 175
Fomitopsis cajanderi 175
Fomitopsis officinalis 155
Fomitopsis pinicola 155
Frost cracks 4
Frost damage 4
Fusarium subglutinans 73

Galls   81, 82
Ganoderma applanatum   178
Ganoderma oregonense   175
Gaseous pollutants   19
Grovesiella canker   75
Grovesiella (Scleroderris) abieticola   75
Gymnosporangium confusum   108
Gymnosporangium cupressi   108
Gymnosporangium fuscum   106
Gymnosporangium harknessianum   106
Gymnosporangium inconspicuum   107
Gymnosporangium kernianum   107
Gymnosporangium libocedri   104
Gymnosporangium multiporum   107
Gymnosporangium nelsonii   108

Hail damage   28
Hawthorn-juniper rust   108
Heat canker   12
Hemlock dwarf mistletoe   133
Herbicide toxicity   18
Hericium abietis   170
Herpotrichia coulteri   34
Herpotrichia juniperi   34
Heterobasidion annosum   137, 138, 166
High temperature   11
High water table   14
Honey mushroom   164
Human activities   29
Hydrogen fluoride damage   23
Hypodermella laricis   36

Ice damage   25
Incense-cedar mistletoe   117
Incense-cedar rust   104
Inconspicuous juniper rust   107
Indian paint fungus   165
Inland spruce cone rust   109
Inonotus tomentosus   174

Juniper mistletoe   117
Juniper pocket rot   168
Juniper rust   107

Knobcone pine dwarf mistletoe   132

Lacquer fungus   175
Laetiporus sulphureus   162
Laminated root rot   172
Larch dwarf mistletoe   128
Larch needle cast   36
Larch needle blight   36
Lentinus lepideus   158
Leptographium wagneri   137, 144
Lightning damage   24
Limber pine dwarf mistletoe   125
Lirula abietis-concoloris   42
Lirula nervisequia var. *conspicua*   44
Lodgepole pine dwarf mistletoe   123
Lodgepole pine needle cast   57
Lophodermella arcuata   50
Lophodermella cerina   54
Lophodermella morbida   55
Lophodermium conigenum   52
Lophodermium crassum   35
Lophodermium decorum   44
Lophodermium juniperi   36
Lophodermium nitens   52
Lophodermium piceae   35
Lophodermium pinastri   52
Lophodermium pini-excelsae   52
Lophodermium seditiosum   52
Low temperature damage   1

Macrophomina phaseolina   149
Mechanical damage   25
Medusa needle blight   57
Melampsora albertensis   102
Melampsora medusae   102
Melampsorella caryophyllacearum   98
Meria laricis   36
Mineral deficiency   17
Mistletoe   4
Mottled rot   172
Mountain hemlock dwarf mistletoe   133
Mycosphaerella pini   48

Necrotic flecks   11
Necrotic canker of white fir   76
Nectria fuckeliana   76
Needle droop   12

Needle scorch 11
Needle tip dieback 16, 17
Nelson's juniper rust 108
Nitrogen deficiency 17

Oligoporus amarus 159
Oligoporus balsameus 175
Oligoporus sequoiae 162
Oyster mushroom 176
Ozone injury 20

Parch blight 10
Particulate pollutants 18
Pear–juniper rust 106
Perenniporia subacida 179
Peridermium filamentosum 91
Peridermium harknessii 92
Peridermium stalactiforme 89
Phacidium abietis 44
Phaeocryptopus gaumannii 39
Phaeolus schweinitzii 147, 160
Phellinus pini 168
Phellinus weirii 137, 146, 171
Pholiota adiposa 172
Phomopsis canker of Douglas fir 70
Phomopsis (Diaporthe) lokoyae 70
Phoradendron densum 115
Phoradendron juniperinum 117
Phoradendron libocedri 117
Phoradendron pauciflorum 115
Phosphorus deficiency 17
Phytophthora cinnamomi 147
Phytophthora lateralis 148
Pinyon dwarf mistletoe 127
Pinyon rust 95
Pitch canker of pines 73
Pleurotus ostreatus 176
Pocket dry rot 159
Pole blight 13
Polyporus amarus 159
Polyporus anceps 176
Polyporus basilaris 175
Polyporus sulphureus 162
Polyporus tomentosus 174
Polyporus volvatus 176

197

Poria albipellucida   174
Poria sequoiae   162
Poria weirii   137, 146, 171
Poria weirii root rot   171
Pouch fungus   176
Pseudomonas pseudotsugae   81
Pucciniastrum epilobii   102
Pucciniastrum goeppertianum   101
Purple discoloration   11
Pyrofomes demidoffii   168

Quinine fungus   155

Red band needle blight   48
Red belt   7
Red belt fungus   155
Red brown butt rot   160
Red ring rot   168
Red root and butt rot   174
Red rot   177
Redwood canker   78
Redwood cubical rot   162
Redwood gall   82
Rhabdocline pseudotsugae   40
Rhabdocline weirii   40
Road salt damage   15
Rotary snow plow damage   15

Salt spray   16
Scaly cap fungus   158
Scleroderris abieticola   75
Sclerophoma pythiophila   74, 80
Sclerophoma canker of pines   74
Sclerophoma tip dieback of fir   80
Seiridium sp.   78
Seiridium (Coryneum) cardinale   77
Serpentine soil   17
Serviceberry rust   107
Sewage effluent   17
Shoestring fungus   164
Shoestring root rot   164
Shoot tip dieback   11
Singleleaf pine needle cast   52
Snow blight   44
Snow damage   25

Soft spongy rot   164
Soil drought   13
Sphaeropsis sapinea   74
Spike top (See top kill)
Spring frost   4
Spruce needle casts   35
Stalactiform rust   89
Sugar pine dwarf mistletoe   122
Sugar pine needle cast   50
Sulfur dioxide   22
Sulfur fungus   162
Sun scorch   7
Sweetfern rust   97
Swiss needle cast   39
Sydowia polyspora   80

Tarweed rust   97
Top kill   4
True fir dwarf mistletoe   122
Twisted needles   18

Uredo cupressicola   109

"Velvet top" fungus   147, 160
Virgella robusta   42

Western dwarf mistletoe   124
Western gall rust   92
Western hemlock dwarf mistletoe   133
Western white pine dwarf mistletoe   131
White fir mistletoe   115
White mottled rot   178
White pine blister rust   85
White pocket rot   168
White ring rot   174
Wind effects   29
   Windthrow   29
   Winter drying (See sun scorch)
   Winter kill   1
   Winter yellows   11

Yellow cap fungus   172
Yellow root rot   179
Yellow pitted rot   170
Yellow witches–broom of fir   98

199